When
Your
Kidneys
Fail

When Your Kidneys Fail

THIRD EDITION

A Handbook for Patients
and Their Families

Mickie Hall Faris, M.P.H., M.B.A.

NKF **National Kidney Foundation ®**
of Southern California
5777 W. Century Blvd., Suite 1450
Los Angeles, California 90045-7404
(310) 641-8152
www.kidneysocal.org

Published and Distributed by the
NATIONAL KIDNEY FOUNDATION
OF
SOUTHERN CALIFORNIA
5777 W Century Blvd., Suite 1450
Los Angeles, California 90045-7404
(310) 641-8152

First Printing, 1982
Revised Edition, 1984
Second Edition, 1987
Revised Second Edition, 1991
Third Edition, 1994

Edited by Carol J. Amato

Library of Congress Catalog Card Number: 87-60180

Printed in the United States of America

To all people
living with chronic kidney failure,
who asked the questions
and inspired us to search
for the answers.

FOREWORD

Kidney failure was one of the most frightening experiences of my life. At one time, before the medical and scientific community developed a method of treatment called "maintenance dialysis," chronic kidney failure was considered fatal.

I have received maintenance dialysis since early 1975 and have undergone two unsuccessful kidney transplant operations. Although I need to make some adjustments to life with kidney failure, I am still able to lead a fairly normal life. One of the most important things that has helped me to adjust has been education about kidney failure and treatment. As a result of this better understanding, I have been able to cope with my illness and enjoy a reasonably happy and productive life.

This third edition has been updated to include the newest information on kidney failure and treatment. I know that this book, which is so easy to read, would have been helpful if I had read it when I first began dialysis.

Donald Hopkins

PREFACE

During my ten-year affiliation with the National Kidney Foundation of Southern California, I have talked with hundreds of people who are facing kidney failure. I have always believed that people receiving treatment for kidney failure are people first and patients second. Treatment becomes a part of one's life, but does not need to become the way of life. Adjustment to kidney failure and treatment can come when anxiety, or the fear of the unknown, is reduced. In this case, the unknown is the lack of information about kidney failure and the treatment that will follow.

When Your Kidneys Fail is a result of many years of thought, discussion with health care professionals and experiences in talking with people who are facing this adjustment in their lives. The handbook is designed to make the information readily available by enabling you to simply look up the particular chapter of interest, find the question and turn to the answer. This handbook can be read either from cover to cover or a section at a time.

The content of this handbook does not include all possible information about kidney failure and treatment. It does, however, provide enough information to help form questions that can be answered by a physician.

Finally, it is not my intent to advocate one method of treatment over another. I have focused on the treatment method known as hemodialysis because, in most cases, it is the initial treatment for people with chronic kidney failure.

M.H.F.

ACKNOWLEDGMENTS

Since the publication of the first edition of *When Your Kidneys Fail*, it has served as a valuable guide for people with chronic kidney failure. Living with this disease requires significant, often profound, adjustments in many aspects of life. Dialysis therapy alters the routine of daily life for people receiving treatment and their families. Dietary restrictions are almost always needed. Transplantation requires, in many cases, the use of potent immuno-suppressant agents that increase the risk of serious infections. The personal economic impact of this disease may be enormous. To deal with the multiple implications of the disease, a team of physicians, nurses, technicians, dietitians and social workers is needed.

Advances in research and in the medical and surgical management of kidney disease led to the need to review and revise this handbook. This task would not have been possible without the important contributions made by the consulting reviewers. With appreciation, we acknowledge the contributions of Mohammad Akmal, M.D.; Arlene Antonoff, L.C.S.W.; Sharon Aronoff; Yolanda Daniele, R.N.; Gabriel Danovitch, M.D.; Barbara Facher, L.C.S.W.; Melissa Heidsman, B.S.W.; Elaine Kamil, M.D.; Gordon Lore; Raimund Hirschberg, M.D.; Rhoda Makoff, Ph.D.; Ronald Miller, M.D.; Glenn Nagami, M.D.; Allen R. Nissenson, M.D.; Mike Paget; Kris Robinson; Paul Serchia; Ruth Sugerman, L.C.S.W.; and Jean Winn, R.N.

The first and second editions of this handbook also reflect the collaborative efforts of many professionals and volunteers. Previous editions were made possible with the support of Charlene G. Brax, M.P.H.; Barbara Bromley, R.N.; Karen Dyer, R.D.; Eben Feinstein, M.D.; David A. Goldstein, M.D.; Donald Hopkins; Ron Husser; Jackie McCreadie; Merlene Pichon, R.D.; Annette James-Rogers, L.C.S.W.; Morris A. Scholl; Michelle Stutz, L.C.S.W.; Sylvie Tarro, M.A.; and A. Tyler Upham, M.D.

RESOURCE ORGANIZATIONS

For Southern California Counties
National Kidney Foundation of Southern California
5777 West Century Boulevard. Suite 1450
Los Angeles, CA 90045-7404
(310) 641-8152

For Northern California Counties
National Kidney Foundation of Northern California
553 Pilgrim Drive, Suite C
Foster City, CA 94404
(650) 349-5111

Other Resources
American Association of Kidney Patients
111 South Parker Street, Suite 405
Tampa. FL 33606
(813) 251-0725
(800) 749-AAKP

National Kidney Foundation, Inc.
30 East 33rd Street, 11th Floor
New York, NY 10016
(800) 622-9010

Southern California Renal Disease Council Network Council #18
6255 Sunset Boulevard, Suite 2211
Hollywood, CA 90028
(213) 962-2020
(800) NEPHROS

Table of Contents

Chapter 7

DIET AND MEDICATION

Chapter 8
ADJUSTMENT AND REHABILITATION

Chapter 9
FINANCIAL INFORMATION AND OTHER RESOURCES

Chapter 10
RESEARCH AND KIDNEY FAILURE

Chapter 12
  ADVANCE DIRECTIVES
  Making Medical Decisions, Limiting Undesired Treatment and Using a Living Will or Durable Power of Attorney to Ensure Your Treatment Preferences Are Respected

When Your Kidneys Fail

Kidney Function 1

The kidneys are organs in the body whose function is necessary to maintain life. Most people are born with two kidneys, located in the middle of the back, one on each side of the spine (see Figure 1).

What are kidneys?

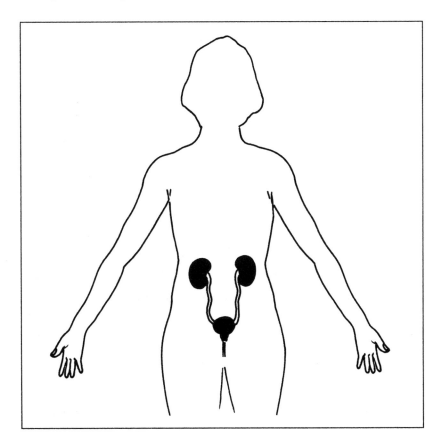

Figure 1.
Location of the kidneys

What is the function of the kidneys?

Most people associate kidneys with urine formation. In making the urine, the kidneys can get rid of extra water, salt and other chemicals that the body does not need. The kidneys also keep water and other substances the body needs from being lost in the urine. The kidneys are the body's "master chemists."

The kidneys have many functions. They:

- adjust the body's fluids
- balance the body's chemicals
- remove waste products from the body
- release several hormones

These functions are described in greater detail in the following paragraphs.

BODY FLUIDS. The kidneys regulate the removal or retention of body fluids. If a person takes in a large amount of salt (sodium) in their diet, they become thirsty and may drink more fluid. If the kidneys are normal, they remove the extra salt and fluid in the urine. If the kidneys are not working properly, the extra salt and fluid build up in the body and may cause the hands, feet and face to swell. This swelling is called edema. If there is too much fluid in the body, it can collect in the lungs and make breathing difficult. It can also put an extra strain on the heart.

BODY CHEMICALS. The normal kidney balances the internal chemistry of the body. The kidneys not only remove certain chemicals, but also keep other substances and chemicals that the body needs. *Potassium* is one of the substances the body needs for normal heart and muscle function. When one

2

eats food with potassium in it, the kidneys work to keep a normal level of potassium in the blood. If the kidneys are not working properly and the potassium builds up in the blood, then muscle function is affected, which may cause weakness. Too much potassium in the blood can also affect the heart, at times, to a dangerous degree. Several chemical reactions in the body produce *acid substances*. Normally, the body maintains a healthy balance of acid. If too many acid substances build up in the body, the kidney responds by adding a buffer to normalize the balance. If the kidney is not working, the normal acid balance cannot be controlled, which can cause a condition called *acidosis*. Normal kidneys also balance other substances in the body that include *protein*. Also, certain kidney diseases result in a leak of protein into the urine, which can even contribute to malnutrition.

WASTE PRODUCTS. Waste products are formed from the breakdown of the protein contained in foods and from normal muscle activity. When the kidneys are not functioning, these waste products build up in the blood and may act like poisons to the body. The buildup of waste products can cause one to be tired, weak and nauseated. This is sometimes called *uremia*, *uremic syndrome* or *uremic poisoning*, because urea is one of the waste products that builds up.

HORMONES. Hormones are substances released by glands and organs to stimulate a specific activity elsewhere in the body. Normal kidneys release several hormones, three of which are *renin*, *erythropoietin* and

3

an activated form of Vitamin D. Renin helps to regulate blood pressure. In non-functioning kidneys, the release of renin can become uncontrollable and can cause high blood pressure. The kidneys release erythropoietin to help the bone marrow make red blood cells. When the kidneys are not working, fewer red blood cells are made, which is a cause of anemia. Activated Vitamin D regulates calcium absorption from food and helps maintain normal bone structure. When kidney function is impaired, less calcium enters the body and bone disease can result.

How do the kidneys function? Blood enters the kidneys through arteries from the heart. The blood is then cleansed as it passes through tiny filters called *nephrons*. The waste products and fluid are filtered out, forming the urine, which is passed through the ureter and then to the bladder. When the bladder is full, the urine is passed out of the body through the urethra (see Figure 2).

Does everyone have two kidneys? No. Some people are born with only one kidney or have lost the function of their second kidney. If the remaining kidney is healthy or functions properly, they can continue to live normal lives. Other people are born with more than two kidneys. These extra kidneys usually do not function.

What are the symptoms of chronic kidney disease? Usually, the first symptom of chronic kidney disease that may cause a person to see a physician is a general feeling of tiredness. However, many symptoms can occur when the kidneys are not working properly. Six of the major warning signs are:

4

- a change in the frequency or pattern of urination
- burning during urination
- bloody or coffee-colored urine
- swelling of the face, feet or abdomen
- lower back pain
- high blood pressure

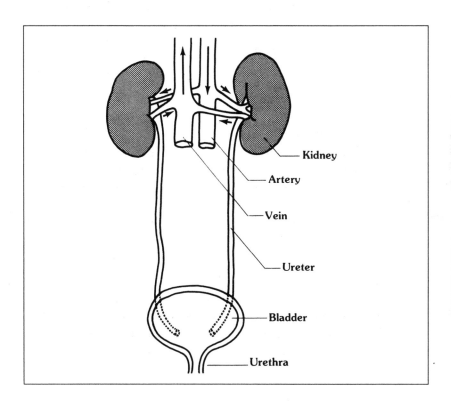

Figure 2.
Kidney function

It is possible that a person may not have these signs even though they are losing kidney function. Very often physical examinations and laboratory tests are needed to detect the problem. Other symptoms of chronic kidney disease are:

- inability to concentrate
- dizziness
- inability to sleep at night
- itchiness all over the body
- decreased appetite, nausea
- an abnormal taste in the mouth
- vomiting
- weight loss
- numbness in arms and legs
- feeling of coldness
- burning sensation in the feet
- headaches
- slurred or mumbled speech

What happens if both kidneys fail?

As kidneys begin to fail, initially, there may be no symptoms. A change in diet and the use of medications may suffice. If both kidneys fail to function, then ongoing medical treatment is needed. This treatment can be either some form of dialysis or kidney transplantation.

What is the difference between acute kidney failure and chronic kidney failure?

The main differences between the two types of kidney failure, acute and chronic, are how quickly the process of kidney failure occurs, the causes of the kidney failure and the duration of the kidney failure.

ACUTE KIDNEY FAILURE is the rapid stopping of kidney function, which can occur during a period of a few hours or days. There are many possible causes of acute kidney failure, which can include severe shock and loss of blood, possibly from an auto accident, burn injury, gunshot wound or extensive surgery; certain types of poisoning; certain types of a

6

kidney disease called *glomerulonephritis*; and injury to or blockage of the blood vessels leading to the kidneys. During the period that the kidneys are not functioning, some form of dialysis may be necessary. Normal kidney function may return after a few weeks to several months, after which dialysis is no longer needed.

CHRONIC KIDNEY FAILURE occurs from the destruction of normal kidney tissues over a longer length of time. Very often there are no symptoms until more than half of the kidney function is lost. When very little kidney function remains, the physician recommends either some form of dialysis or kidney transplantation to maintain life. The kidney function in chronic kidney failure does not return except in very rare instances.

What is the treatment for kidney failure?

As kidney function is lost, a physician may recommend drugs to control high blood pressure and a special diet low in protein to reduce the level of toxins in the body. When this treatment is no longer effective and there is very little kidney function remaining, either some form of dialysis or kidney transplantation becomes necessary for survival. These should be considered months in advance of the symptoms of kidney failure so that there is time to consider which form of treatment is most suitable and least inconvenient for a person, and to prepare for dialysis or transplantation. Rarely do people elect to forgo such treatment because they judge the burdens of other non-kidney illnesses (which are not benefited by dialysis or transplantation) outweigh the benefits of surviving on dialysis or having kidney function restored by a transplant.

What are the causes of chronic kidney failure?

Chronic kidney failure has many possible causes, some of which are:

- some forms of diabetes, which can create a condition called diabetic *nephropathy*

- hypertension, or high blood pressure, which can damage the blood vessels in the kidney and reduce the blood supply to the kidney, thereby causing a condition called *nephrosclerosis*

- *chronic glomerulonephritis*, which results from an inflammation in the kidney that destroys kidney tissue

- *polycystic kidney disease*, an inherited disease, which causes the normal kidney tissue to be replaced by cysts

- *pyelonephritis*, which is a chronic infection of the kidney

- *interstitial nephritis*, which is a chronic inflammation of the kidney, sometimes due to certain drugs

- *systemic lupus erythematosus* (SLE), a connective tissue disorder, which may affect many organs in the body

- *arteriosclerosis*, or hardening of the arteries

There are other possible causes of kidney failure besides the ones mentioned. For more information on those, as well as more information on the ones listed, a person should talk to their physician.

What is End-Stage Renal Disease (ESRD)?

End-Stage Renal Disease (ESRD) has the same meaning as the term *irreversible chronic kidney failure*, or that stage of kidney damage requiring dialysis or kidney transplantation. Physicians and other health care professionals often use the term *ESRD*.

When is dialysis or kidney transplantation needed?

When kidney function is reduced to approximately five percent of normal, or when 95 percent function has been lost, either some form of dialysis or kidney transplantation is needed to maintain life. The percentage of remaining function below which treatment is required may vary with the individual depending upon the person's health and their physician's recommendation.

Methods of Treatment 2

Dialysis is a form of medical treatment that removes the body's wastes directly from the blood of people who have lost kidney function. Dialysis replaces some of the functions that the kidneys can no longer perform. There are two forms of dialysis: *hemodialysis* (also called *artificial kidney treatment*) and *peritoneal dialysis.*

What is dialysis?

Hemodialysis is a form of dialysis that uses an artificial kidney machine (dialysis machine) to remove fluids and waste products from the bloodstream. An access is usually placed in the arm or leg, and blood is taken from the access usually through a needle inserted into the artery end of the access. A tube is attached to the needle and carries blood to the dialysis machine. The heart pumps blood with the assistance of a blood pump through the tube to the machine, where it is cleansed by running through a dialyzer (artificial kidney) and returned to the body through a tube and then through a needle that has been inserted into the vein end of the access. The blood is continuously circulated; only about a pint is outside the body at a time through the dialyzer until the treatment has been completed. Hemodialysis is explained in greater detail in Chapter 3.

What is hemodialysis?

Peritoneal dialysis is another method of removing waste, extra salt and fluid from the body. However, instead of using an artificial

What is peritoneal dialysis?

11

kidney, as in hemodialysis, the lining of the abdominal cavity is used. A peritoneal dialysis catheter is surgically implanted in the abdomen, usually below the navel. A specially prepared solution called peritoneal dialysate is dripped into the abdomen through the catheter. After a specified length of time, the used dialysate is allowed to flow out of the abdominal cavity through the catheter. After it has drained, fresh dialysate is sent back in and the procedure is repeated. This procedure, known as a solution exchange, is repeated several times a day. See Chapter 4 for additional information.

What is kidney transplantation?

Another major treatment for kidney failure is kidney transplantation. This involves removing a kidney from either a living relative or from an unrelated deceased person and surgically placing the new kidney into the patient. See Chapter 5 for additional information. Today, non-related living donors may be used if there is the proper tissue matching.

When was dialysis treatment developed?

The first modern artificial kidney was successfully developed during World War II by Dr. Willem Kolff in Holland. Until the 1960s, it was used only for short periods of time for acute kidney failure. Dr. Belding Scribner developed a special access device in 1960, called a Scribner shunt, which made it possible to perform repeated treatments indefinitely for chronic kidney failure.

Does dialysis cure chronic kidney failure?

No. Dialysis or artificial kidney treatment does not cure chronic kidney failure, but it does allow a person to maintain life and reasonable health.

Hemodialysis 3

Artificial kidney treatment performs the most critical of the vital functions that the normal kidney does. First, the artificial kidney helps to maintain fluid balance by removing excess fluid from the body through a process called *ultrafiltration*. Second, the artificial kidney removes waste products and balances potentially toxic chemicals in the blood, through a process known as *diffusion*. By combining ultrafiltration and diffusion, the artificial kidney balances the fluid and chemicals in the body and excretes important waste products.

How does hemodialysis work?

The artificial kidney, or dialyzer, is made up of two compartments. The blood flows to the first compartment, called the blood compartment, where it then flows within a semipermeable membrane, outside of which is the dialysate compartment. The dialysate compartment holds the clear dialysate solution necessary for the removal of waste products, and that allows chemical balance to take place. The membrane in the dialyzer prevents the blood from mixing together with the dialysate solution and allows for ultrafiltration for fluid balance, diffusion for chemical balance and removal of waste products through submicroscopic holes in the membrane. These same holes allow certain molecules or substances to move through and across the membrane, but they are too small to allow red and white blood cells, proteins and bacteria to cross through. Figure 3 shows the hemodialysis process.

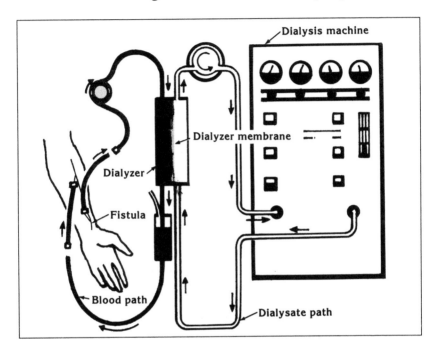

Figure 3.
The hemodialysis process

ULTRAFILTRATION is the dialysis process that removes fluids from the blood. Ultrafiltration occurs because of negative pressure exerted by a vacuum pump in the dialysate circuit that pulls fluid out of the blood. Figure 4 shows an example of ultrafiltration. Ultrafiltration uses a positive pressure on the blood side of the dialysis membrane, which accomplishes the same thing (removal of the extra fluid from the blood and body) as the negative pressure on the dialysate side of the membrane.

DIFFUSION is the process that allows the passage of chemicals and fluids through the semipermeable membrane of the dialyzer. When two solutions of different concentrations are separated by a semipermeable membrane, such as the one in a dialyzer, very small particles or molecules in the two solutions move back and forth across the membrane to make the two solutions equal in concentration, if the molecules are small and the process is allowed to continue for some time. The molecules may move from solution A to solution B or from solution B to solution A. This movement of molecules back and forth through the membrane is called diffusion. Figure 5 shows an example of diffusion using a solution A (salt solution) and a solution B (pure water). During dialysis, the blood and the dialysate are the two solutions of different concentrations, separated by the membrane. The blood contains a high concentration of waste products. Because the dialysate does not contain any waste products, they transfer across the membrane from the blood into the dialysate. The dialysate contains chemicals, such as potassium, but at lower levels than the blood, allowing some of the extra potassium in the body to transfer from the blood into the dialysate. Dialysate also contains a substance called *acetate* (which is not contained in the blood) or *bicarbonate* (which is in the body in lower concentrations than in the dialysate). Because there is no acetate and less bicarbonate in the blood than in the dialysate, the substances transfer from the dialysate into the blood to help maintain the acid-base balance.

15

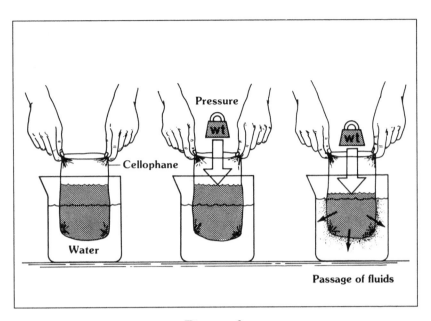

Figure 4.
Ultrafiltration

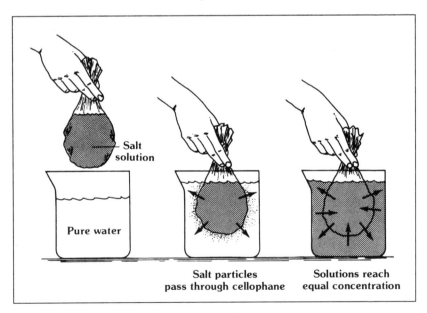

Figure 5.
Diffusion

Yes. Dialyzer and artificial kidney mean the same thing. Both terms refer to that part of the hemodialysis system that contains the membrane (which filters the blood), and has blood and dialysate compartments.

Do dialyzer and artificial kidney have the same meaning?

Hemodialysis is the most frequently used form of dialysis in the United States. The determination whether to initiate hemodialysis treatment rather than peritoneal dialysis (or transplantation rather than either form of dialysis treatment) is based on health, the cause of kidney failure, age, lifestyle, the availability of a suitable kidney donor, and, of course, personal preference and other factors.

Do physicians recommend hemodialysis over other forms of treatment?

Yes. The decision of which type of treatment to choose should be a combined decision involving you, your family, a physician and other health care personnel. While you can decide which treatment is most suitable to fit your work and personal lifestyle, a physician recommends which treatment best meets your medical needs. The combined input should decide the treatment of choice.

Do I have a choice in selecting treatment?

A person requires dialysis two or three times a week, unless it is done continuously or nightly via the peritoneum. A physician determines how often dialysis is needed, as well as the duration of each treatment.

How often is hemodialysis treatment needed?

High-flux hemodialysis is a technique that speeds up dialysis using a very permeable dialyzer and a special dialysis machine. Another important aspect of this technique is

What is high-flux hemodialysis?

17

the use of bicarbonate rather than acetate in the dialysate solution, which helps to reduce some side effects and enables a person to tolerate the treatment better. Since this technique requires special equipment, it is not available at all dialysis centers. In addition, a person may not be a good candidate for this technique and should discuss it with their physician. High-flux dialysis is highly efficient and usually allows shorter dialysis treatments. Somewhat shorter treatments can also be achieved using conventional membranes and much faster blood flows. This technique is sometimes called *high-efficiency dialysis.*

Where do I go to get hemodialysis treatment?

Hemodialysis centers are located throughout the United States. Most people today receive their treatment in a full-care outpatient facility. These centers can be located either in a hospital or outside of a hospital. Also, with special training, you can dialyze in your own home. A list of dialysis centers is available from the National Kidney Foundation affiliate. A physician is the best person to talk to about where to go for dialysis treatment. The Nephrology Resource Directory also contains a fairly complete listing of all the ESRD facilities in the U.S.

Do all centers have the same dialysis schedule?

No. The dialysis treatment schedules vary with each center. Most centers have one or two shifts to provide treatment during the daytime hours. Other facilities also have evening and Saturday shifts to provide treatment for people who work.

A nurse or trained technician takes care of the procedures of putting you on the artificial kidney machine and taking you off when you receive treatment in a hospital or in a full-care facility. The nurse or technician connects the bloodstream access line to the machine, monitors the system during the run and disconnects the blood lines after the treatment is completed. If the treatment is performed in the home, you and another trained person perform the necessary procedure.

How are the hemodialysis treatments done? Who does them?

Monitors are devices that measure several dialysis functions during treatment. Their purpose is to provide safe dialysis treatment and to respond with a light and a noise to alert the staff when something is wrong. When a monitor indicates an alarm, dialysis may be automatically stopped. In most cases, the problem is not immediately dangerous to you and can be quickly corrected by the staff. The combination of the monitors and the supervision of the staff helps to make dialysis treatment safe and comfortable. The *venous pressure monitor* and the *arterial pressure monitor* measure the pressure of the blood as it flows through the dialyzer. If there is a break, kink or any obstruction in the blood lines or in the dialyzer, the pressure changes and the monitors send out an alarm to alert you and the staff. The *temperature monitor* indicates an alarm if the dialysate solution is too hot or too cold. Because the blood normally cools when it leaves the body through the blood lines, it must be rewarmed to the normal body temperature before it is returned to the body. This is accomplished by heating

Why are monitors needed and what do they do?

19

the dialysate solution, which, in turn, rewarms the blood. The *negative pressure monitor* shows the amount of suction or negative pressure used to remove the excess fluid from the body. An alarm sounds if this pressure changes. Another very important device on the artificial kidney machine is the *blood leak monitor*, which sets off an alarm if any blood leaks into the dialysate solution through a tear in the dialyzer membrane. The *conductivity monitor* indicates the concentration of substances in the dialysate solution. The *air detector* detects any air or foam that might pass through the system. This detector not only indicates an alarm, but also has an automatic device that clamps the blood line returning to the body to prevent air from being pushed into the vein. It may be frightening when an alarm sounds, but the monitors are designed to protect you and to make treatment as safe and comfortable as possible.

What is the blood flow rate?

This is the rate at which blood flows through the dialyzer.

Is the artificial kidney or dialyzer used more than once?

Some centers clean and resterilize their dialyzers and use them again. Other centers use them once and then discard them. When dialyzers are used more than once, they are carefully marked and stored and used again only for the same patient. They are tested to be sure they function adequately (and in some respects may be better than a new dialyzer).

Hemodialysis treatment is essentially pain-less; however, depending on what type of access device you have, you may feel slight discomfort when the needle is placed in the skin. You may also have occasional nausea, headaches or muscle cramps during treatment.

Does hemodialysis treatment hurt?

Most people require two-and-one-half to five hours of treatment. The length of a treatment depends on your body size; the intake of fluid, protein, potassium, and other nutrients between dialysis; the type of dialyzer used; the type of equipment used; the blood flow achievable through the access; and the remaining kidney function.

How long does the treatment take?

Each person responds differently to dialysis, although many people actually feel better after they begin receiving dialysis treatments. Because dialysis cannot replace the loss of *erythropoietin*, the hormone that helps to make red blood cells, you may become anemic and tired as a result. In the past, when this was the case, a physician could prescribe medication to help build up the number of red blood cells, but often, transfusions were necessary. Now genetically engineered erythropoietin is available, and transfusions are needed only when there is bleeding or sudden blood loss.

Will I be tired all the time?

The way you feel will depend on your health and how much uremic poison and fluid is in your system. You may feel somewhat tired immediately after a treatment. One way to work on feeling well is for you to adhere to the prescribed diet, medications and fluid

How will I feel before, during, and after treatment?

allowances between treatments. Excessive fluid intake can cause heart failure and severe shortness of breath.

What can I do during treatment?
You can read, watch television, do paperwork, conduct business over the phone or perform other activities. Sleeping is also an option, although you may prefer to stay awake to help monitor the treatment.

Will I be able to urinate?
Some people receiving dialysis treatment can produce only small amounts of urine, others produce normal amounts of urine (though of poor quality), and still others cannot produce any urine. Even if you produce a normal volume of urine, you still need dialysis, because the amount of waste products in your urine is low and continues to build up in the blood.

How long will it take to become adjusted to dialysis?
Much of the anxiety and fear you may experience is because the dialysis treatment is so new and seems very complex at first. Once you become familiar with the treatment, then adjustment can begin. You will not change simply because you are receiving dialysis treatment. If you had difficulty adjusting to other problems in life prior to kidney failure, then it may take a while longer to become comfortable with the treatment. On the other hand, if you adjusted to problems fairly easily prior to dialysis, the adjustment should come more quickly.

Today, there are over 170,000 people being treated with artificial kidney treatment in the United States alone.

How many people receive dialysis treatment?

There are people in the United States who have been receiving treatment for over 20 years. No one can tell you how long you will live on dialysis. If you have had no medical problems other than kidney failure, you should have a longer life expectancy than someone who has other chronic medical problems in addition to kidney failure and the need to receive dialysis treatment.

How long can I live while receiving dialysis treatment?

Yes. There are many different types of hemodialysis machines, manufactured by several companies. The various machines may differ in price and appearance; some are more suitable for center use than home use.

Is there more than one type of hemodialysis machine?

The major types of dialyzers used today are the *parallel flow dialyzer* and *capillary dialyzer*. Although each dialyzer operates on the same basic principle, your physician may recommend one type over another.

What are the different types of dialyzers?

To use the artificial kidney, the blood must be passed through the dialyzer, where the waste products and excess fluids are removed, and must be returned to the body. There are three methods of getting blood from the body to the hemodialysis machine and back to the body again. These are the internal fistula, the internal graft and the external shunt or catheter. To be implanted, each device requires surgery.

What are access devices and why are they needed?

23

A physician will recommend which type of access device is best.

What is a fistula? A fistula is created surgically by directly connecting one of the arteries to one of the veins. It is constructed by a surgical procedure under local anesthesia and lies completely under the skin, usually near the wrist or the elbow. Arteries are located deep under the skin and have a fast pulsating flow. Normally, the veins are smaller than the arteries. By joining them, the blood from the artery flows directly to the vein, and the vein becomes larger and is called a "fistula." This makes the insertion of the two needles required for dialysis much easier. During dialysis, a member of the nursing or technician staff cleans the area overlying the internal fistula. The skin may be numbed with a local anesthetic, and two needles are inserted into the vessels, one in the artery portion of the fistula to take blood from you to the dialyzer and one in the vein portion of the fistula to return the blood from the artificial kidney to you (see Figure 6). The needles are attached to tubes that carry the blood to the dialyzer and then back to the body. After the vascular surgeon creates the internal fistula, it often takes several weeks for the veins to become large enough for the needles to enter them easily. The doctor may give you instructions on how to help the veins enlarge so they can be used. Fistulas can clot or become infected, but do so infrequently. Signs of clotting can include disappearance of the vein's pulsation; the sound of blood moving through the vessels; pain; and swelling. Signs of infection include redness, swelling and fever. You should contact your physician if this happens.

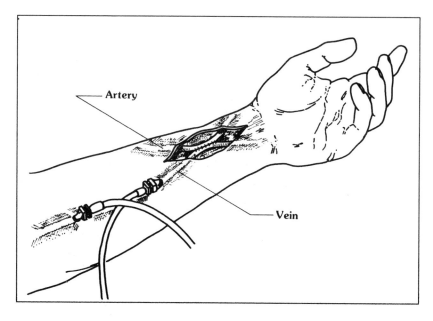

Figure 6.
Internal fistula

What is a graft?

Internal grafts are access devices that are very similar to fistulas, but instead of directly connecting an artery directly to a vein, a tube of synthetic material (a conduit) is inserted to connect the two together.

Do I have to go to a hospital to get dialysis treatment?

If you require a very great deal of care because of a medical complication, or if you need to be hospitalized for a medical or surgical condition, you may need to be dialyzed as an inpatient at a hospital. Dialysis offered in this way is called *inpatient dialysis. Outpatient dialysis* refers to dialysis performed in a facility located outside of a hospital. It may also refer to dialysis performed in a facility located inside a hospital where there are no other medical complications and overnight stay is not needed. During outpatient dialysis, often called *full-care dialysis*, the medical staff performs the dialysis procedure, and after treatment, you are allowed to go home. Another alternative to the hospital-based center is dialysis at home. *Home dialysis* requires special training, and for hemodialysis, the assistance of a family member or friend. Peritoneal dialysis can often be performed by you alone after training. The decision of whether or not you require hospital inpatient dialysis should be left to your physician. Once you are well enough for outpatient dialysis, you can decide, along with the assistance of a physician, whether to try a hospital-based outpatient center, a freestanding (located outside of a hospital) outpatient center or home dialysis.

What is a satellite center? A satellite center is a dialysis center located outside of a hospital but affiliated with a hospital. The term can also be used to refer to a rural dialysis facility at a distance from a supervising dialysis center.

Can I dialyze at home? In order to be able to dialyze at home, you should have a physician's support, which is based on your medical condition. Also, you must have a trained person in attendance to help you with the procedure if you plan to do hemodialysis. Other considerations are:

- adequate room for the equipment and storage of supplies
- access to electricity and drainage
- good water supply

If a family member is involved, their support should be included in the decision.

The training for home dialysis required for you (and for any person who is going to assist) involves teaching you every aspect of your own care while on dialysis. In addition to being taught about diet and medications, you are taught how to:

- prepare the dialysis machine
- put yourself on
- monitor yourself during treatment
- take yourself off
- clean or "tear down" the dialysis machine after treatment has been completed

The length of training for home dialysis varies with the training center, although most training sessions last from one to two months for hemodialysis and a shorter time for peritoneal dialysis.

As with other treatment modalities, there are pros and cons to home dialysis. The pros include:

- more flexibility in scheduling treatment and time saved in the travel to and from the dialysis center
- a better understanding of the treatment procedure
- more time to spend with your family and in the home atmosphere
- more privacy than can be offered in the dialysis center

The cons to home dialysis can include:

- requiring someone trained to assist you (some companies provide a trained assistant as part of their home dialysis service)

- the inability to become trained to do your own self-care safely
- lack of adequate space to accommodate the necessary equipment
- having the equipment in the home as a constant reminder of your need for treatment
- possible added stress to family members

The decision of whether or not to dialyze at home is an individual one. You may prefer being dialyzed by trained professionals in a center, or you may enjoy the freedom of being able to dialyze at home.

What is the difference between full-care and self-care dialysis?

If you choose full-care dialysis, you dialyze in an outpatient dialysis center and the treatment is administered by the dialysis staff. If you have self-care dialysis at home or in a special self-care center (of which there are relatively few nowadays), you are responsible for most of your own care with the assistance of another trained individual (such as a spouse at home or a nurse or technician who may oversee the care of many patients in a self-care center).

Which dialysis location is best?

No dialysis location is considered best for all people. The decision to dialyze at a facility or at home should be made with the assistance of a physician.

Are there risks in hemodialysis?

Yes, as there are for virtually any treatment. Dialysis is a complicated procedure that must be done carefully to assure safety. The highly trained professionals, along with the safety features of dialysis machines, work together to keep the risks to a minimum.

Although some problems can occur during hemodialysis, most of them can be prevented or solved. These problems can include blood leaks, incorrect dialysis concentrate, infection and hypotension, which is low blood pressure.

What are the possible medical problems that can occur during hemodialysis?

The membrane of the dialyzer can develop a small leak and, on rare occasions, a larger break. If this happens, blood leaks from the blood compartment into the dialysate. A monitor detects this immediately and sends off an alarm, and the tubes connecting you to the dialyzer are temporarily closed off until the dialyzer membrane is replaced. Another type of blood leak can occur in the tubes carrying the blood between you and the dialyzer. A pressure monitor sends out an alarm and the problem is corrected at once.

What are blood leaks?

Concentrated dialysate is mixed with precisely the correct amount of water to produce dialysate for hemodialysis. If the dialysis concentrate is mixed incorrectly, you may have immediate side effects, such as vomiting and muscle ache. Most dialysis machines are equipped with monitors that send out alarms if the concentrate is incorrect. For peritoneal dialysis, concentrates are not used nowadays.

Is the dialysis concentrate important?

29

Are there different types of dialysis concentrate?

Yes. The two most common types of concentrate are acetate and bicarbonate dialysate. Bicarbonate dialysate is commonly used today because of fewer side effects.

Are there different types of peritoneal dialysate?

Yes. The most common difference is the amount of glucose (sugar) in the dialysate. Higher concentrations of glucose help to remove more fluid from the body and are used when necessary to achieve fluid balance.

Can I get an infection because of dialysis treatment?

In most cases, infection from dialysis can be avoided by using proper sterile techniques, which include the proper cleansing of the skin and the application of an antiseptic to any point of needle entry or opening of the blood lines. The risk of infection is greater if you have an external device (a shunt or a subclavian or peritoneal catheter) rather than an internal fistula.

Is hepatitis common?

Hepatitis is a viral infection of the liver. In most cases, it causes a short-term illness that gradually clears up over a period of two or three weeks. However, in some cases, hepatitis leads to chronic infection that causes serious liver damage. Hepatitis C is a form of viral hepatitis that is transmitted primarily by the transfer of blood or blood products from one individual to another. It is being found more frequently in dialysis centers due to increased awareness of its existence and the availability of a test to detect it.

Another form of hepatitis, serum hepatitis, or Hepatitis B, may also occur in people on dialysis. The most common way that serum hepatitis spreads is through contact with blood. People receiving dialysis treatment are at a higher risk of acquiring Hepatitis C and (serum) Hepatitis B than others because of the nature of the treatment, possible contact with an infected needle (which should not occur) and because of blood transfusions. A test, known as the Hepatitis B Antigen test, determines who is infected with serum hepatitis. The spread of Hepatitis C and serum hepatitis may be prevented when the dialysis staff members practice universal precautions, as recommended by the Centers for Disease Control and Prevention (CDC), and when they isolate patients known to have a positive Hepatitis B Antigen test or abnormal liver enzymes. In addition, a Hepatitis B vaccine is available that is very effective in preventing infection with serum hepatitis.

What about HIV/AIDS?

AIDS (acquired immune deficiency syndrome) is caused by a virus (Human Immunodeficiency Virus (HIV) and can be carried through blood. It is spread through intimate sexual contact and occasionally through blood products. The spread of this virus through blood products is very uncommon since all blood donors are now tested for HIV antibodies and since the number of viral particles in blood is far less than in Hepatitis B. As in hepatitis, the spread of HIV may be prevented through strict adherence to universal precautions as recommended by the CDC. Dialysis units and dialysis staff are familiar with the essential precautions.

31

What does hypotension mean?

Hypotension is abnormally low blood pressure. Hypotension may be caused by blood leakage or from excess fluid removal during dialysis. If you have hypotension, you can feel faint. The dialysis staff can quickly solve the problem by adding a salt solution (saline) to the bloodstream.

Are there any other medical problems that can occur?

Artificial kidney treatment can and does correct many of the physical problems that result from loss of kidney function and the onset of uremia. However, artificial kidney treatment does not totally replace the function of normal kidneys. Although you may experience long-term complications because of the loss of kidney function, many of these complications can be treated with medication, a change in the dialysis program or possible surgery.

What is fluid overload?

Because the kidneys can no longer remove excess sodium and fluid from the body, dialysis must remove the sodium and fluid entering the body in the diet. If you ingest (take in) too much sodium and fluid between dialysis treatments, you may contract a condition called *fluid overload*. Fluid overload is evident from weight gain and, often, other symptoms, such as difficulty in breathing or shortness of breath and swelling of the ankles. Fluid overload places a strain on the heart because it has to pump more blood than usual. If fluid overload occurs, the treatment can include restricting sodium and fluid intake; either longer or more efficient dialytic ultrafiltration to remove the excess fluid and sodium; careful monitoring of your blood pressure; and possibly medication to lower your blood pressure.

32

Most people on dialysis are anemic because there are too few red blood cells in the body due to the kidney failure. This can be effectively treated with erythropoietin (EPO). See Chapter 5 for more information.

Will I become anemic?

Hyperkalemia means that there is a high level of potassium in the blood. Like sodium and fluid, potassium can also build up in the blood when the kidneys do not function. Potassium enters the body through the diet and hyperkalemia can be avoided by not eating foods high in potassium. There are very few symptoms in hyperkalemia, but when they do appear, they can be serious. These can include an irregular heartbeat and muscular weakness, which would require immediate medical care. The best way to avoid hyperkalemia is for you to be aware of those foods and salt substitutes that are very high in potassium and avoid them.

What does hyperkalemia mean?

Most people with kidney failure have some degree of hypertension or high blood pressure. In some cases, the hypertension may have caused the kidney failure. In other cases, hypertension is a result of damaged kidneys and the release of certain hormones (like renin) into the bloodstream. Your blood pressure can be lowered through use of a wide variety of medications and through the removal of excess fluid from the body during dialysis.

What is hypertension?

Bone disease is a medical problem that affects most people with kidney failure. There are two major types of bone disease: *parathyroid hormone bone disease* and *aluminum bone disease.*

Does bone disease affect all people with kidney disease?

33

Parathyroid hormone bone disease: With kidney failure, the calcium level in the blood may drop. When the calcium decreases in the blood, a reaction in the body is triggered resulting in the release of calcium from the bones. This reaction is caused partially by the parathyroid glands, which are tiny glands located in the neck. The calcium from the bones then goes into the bloodstream to increase the blood calcium level toward normal. The release of calcium from bones may cause them to weaken and may result in bone pain and fractures (broken bones). To keep the calcium and phosphorus levels normal, a physician may prescribe calcium supplements and calcium salts or rarely antacid therapy as phosphate binders. If the calcium level remains low, a physician may prescribe a hormone/vitamin called Vitamin D or *calcitriol*.

Aluminum bone disease: This type of bone disease is caused by a buildup of aluminum in the body, which may prevent normal bone formation. A biopsy of the bone is required to diagnose this disease. Aluminum bone disease can be prevented by reducing the intake of aluminum in the diet and by restricting medications containing aluminum. Treatment of aluminum bone disease may require a regimen of medication called *chelation therapy*.

Are the parathyroid glands ever removed? Yes. Sometimes, the parathyroid glands remain overactive in their attempt to release calcium from the bone and, in doing so, raise the blood calcium level of the blood. If these glands remain overactive for a long time, they can enlarge. When they become larger, they also become more active in releasing hormones and triggering calcium to be removed from the bones. If the parathyroid glands are abnormally overactive, they can be treated with Rocaltral (an active Vitamin D preparation) by mouth and, in some severe cases, intravenously. Surgical removal is rarely performed, but this is done in patients with severe disease and when hyperparathyroidism is resistant to medical treatment, including Vitamin D therapy.

What is neuropathy?

Neuropathy, or nerve damage, may occur because the kidneys have failed. Although the cause of neuropathy is not fully understood, it may be related to the buildup of waste products in the blood, which may cause damage to the nerves and a change in the feeling in the feet, legs or hands. Sometimes, numbness, tingling (sensory neuropathy) or muscular weakness (motion neuropathy) can occur, resulting in decreased sensitivity to temperature and pain. Neuropathy is more common and often more severe if you have diabetes.

Are there other complications?

Yes. Restlessness and almost involuntary movement of the legs are symptoms that you may experience. A person may find that sleeping with a bed partner is no longer possible. The physician should be notified if this problem exists. Very often, this problem is caused by insufficient dialysis.

What kind of medications will I need during hemodialysis treatment? The most common medications required during dialysis are *anticoagulants*, which are used to prevent the blood from clotting in the artificial kidney and the blood lines to and from it. Blood clots, in turn, could cause the blood line to become blocked.

What is heparinization? *Heparin* is a drug or anticoagulant that prevents the blood from clotting during dialysis treatment. *Heparinization* is the procedure by which you receive heparin during dialysis. In this method, heparin is added to the blood as it leaves the body. Heparinization may require a special pump called a heparin pump. By the end of dialysis, the effect of the heparin begins to wear off and blood clotting becomes normal.

Why do I need blood studies? Blood studies are usually performed to determine if you are maintaining your diet and medication properly and also to evaluate the effectiveness of your dialysis treatment. A group of blood tests is usually done monthly as a monitoring method to watch your blood chemistries. Blood may be drawn from the blood tubing at the beginning of a dialysis treatment for laboratory studies and sometimes during and at the end of dialysis. These tests include creatinine, blood urea nitrogen and hematocrit. Other blood tests are performed to determine the levels of potassium, sodium, bicarbonate, calcium and phosphate in the bloodstream. See Appendix A for a table of commonly performed blood tests, including the type of test, the reason for the test and an abbreviation of the test.

Properly functioning kidneys prevent the fluid in the body from building up by removing the excess body fluid as urine. When your kidneys are not functioning, fluid may accumulate in your bloodstream. A large amount of fluid in your blood can cause high blood pressure and places a strain on your heart. Although fluid can also collect in your lungs, making it hard to breathe, this can be controlled by bringing the body to a dry weight or a weight at which the blood pressure is normal and no swelling is present. You should achieve proper fluid balance by watching your diet and fluid intake between dialysis treatments.

Why is fluid a problem?

Muscle cramps are most likely to occur if you are overweight because of too much fluid in your body. A major cause of muscle cramps is the removal of a large amount of fluid during treatment. The best way to avoid muscle cramps is to limit salt and fluid intake.

Will I have muscle cramps?

You may experience some itching as a result of kidney failure (uremia), the level of phosphorus in the body or allergies to medications you are taking. If the itching symptoms are related to uremia, your physician may increase dialysis or prescribe medications, and, in some cases, recommend ultraviolet light treatments. Your physician adjusts the intake of phosphorus through diet and medication if the itching is related to phosphorus. Your medications may be adjusted if the itching is a result of an allergic reaction to medications.

Is itching a problem?

37

What is creatinine? Creatinine is a byproduct of normal muscle metabolism. Creatinine is removed by the normal kidney, but must be removed by dialysis when your kidneys are not working. Creatinine levels can show if you are taking in enough protein and nutrients to maintain your body's muscle mass as well as indicate the adequacy of dialysis. High levels are not incompatible with health.

What is blood urea nitrogen (BUN)? A test for blood urea nitrogen, or BUN, determines the level of urea in the blood. This test, like the creatinine test, helps determine how effective the dialysis treatments are. Urea comes from the breakdown of protein in the body. Because urea cannot be removed from the body by your kidneys, it and other protein waste products can build up and cause you to become sick. This is why protein in your diet may be restricted. Hemodialysis can more effectively control the body urea when dietary protein intake is limited. This is rarely necessary in peritoneal dialysis, and people on peritoneal dialysis may even be required to increase their protein intake.

What does hematocrit mean? *Hematocrit*, or HCT, is a measure of the number of red blood cells in your blood, specifically the percentage of the blood that is red cells—that is, the percentage of blood that is not serum. The loss of kidney function causes a lower number of red blood cells in the body, which can cause you to become anemic. The hematocrit test monitors the level of blood cells and can alert a physician if medication or a blood transfusion is needed.

If you are severely anemic and experiencing symptoms, you may require a blood transfusion, particularly if you have internal bleeding (as from an ulcer).

Will I need blood transfusions?

Yes. In the dialysis unit, there is a team approach to providing treatment. Each individual on this team contributes their unique professional and personal skills to increase the effectiveness of care. One of the most important members of this team is you. You need to take a great deal of responsibility in your own care. This includes understanding and complying with your diet and medication regimen; noting and reporting unusual symptoms to your physician; and cooperating with other members of the team. The other team members include the physicians, the nursing staff, the technicians, the social worker and the dietitian.

Is there a team approach to providing dialysis treatment?

You may receive care from more than one physician in the dialysis unit. These physicians have received special training in nephrology, which includes studies and clinical experience in the areas of kidney disease, kidney failure and treatment. A physician with this special training is called a nephrologist, or sometimes, a renologist. He or she is also a fully trained internist. Your physician will be responsible for monitoring your physical condition, laboratory tests, and dialysis records to determine the effectiveness of your treatment and whether any other medical complications are taking place, and in general, to supervise your overall medical treatment, health and well-being.

How will a physician take care of me?

39

What is the role of the nursing and technician staff?

Dialysis nurses and patient-care technicians must have special training in order to supervise and perform the technical aspect of dialysis treatment. The specially trained dialysis nurse is capable and qualified to monitor the whole dialysis procedure, which involves supervising the dialysis treatments, starting and discontinuing treatments and initiating any emergency measure that may be required. The staff also includes trained technicians to assist, under the nurses' supervision, in the dialysis treatment. Other technicians set up and maintain the dialysis machines and other equipment.

How can the social worker help?

The social worker is a professional member of the health care team who is trained to help you and your family adjust to the possible day-to-day changes in lifestyle as a result of kidney failure, dialysis treatment and other illnesses. The social worker offers counseling services and resource and referral services. Examples of problems that may benefit from counseling services are depression, anxiety, marital and family stress and sexual concerns. Examples of problems that may require resource and referral services are:

- inability to pay for the cost of dialysis and transplantation, hospital, doctor and pharmacy bills
- insufficient income to meet day-to-day needs
- lack of transportation for travel to and from dialysis treatments
- loss of employment

A dietitian has professional training in dietetics and nutrition and is a specialist in planning meals that have the kinds and quantities of foods and fluids required for special medical needs. Sometimes, dietitians are called nutritionists. The dietitian's main function is to determine any specific nutritional needs and to develop a special diet plan, with supplements, if indicated, tailored to your needs. The dietitian can also provide you and your family with counseling on the importance of diet, menus, food selection, fluid restriction and ways to adjust to your new dietary plan. Many dietitians will review your monthly blood tests with you, since the tests relate to diet as well as to dialysis.

Can a dietitian help me with my diet?

Peritoneal Dialysis

Peritoneal dialysis is a form of dialysis that uses the lining of the abdominal cavity called the *peritoneum* to filter out waste products. A specially prepared solution called peritoneal dialysate is infused (sent) into the abdomen through a catheter inserted into the abdominal cavity. The dialysate is allowed to dwell for a period of time, during which waste products and other substances in excessive concentrates in the blood diffuse across the peritoneal membrane from the body into the dialysate. After the dwell, the dialysate is drained from the body and discarded.

What is peritoneal dialysis?

A peritoneal dialysis catheter or soft plastic tube is surgically placed into the abdomen, often about an inch below the navel. A few inches of this tube remain securely in place outside the body; the other end stays in the abdominal cavity. The peritoneum is used as the dialyzing surface or membrane. A drawing of the catheter as it is placed in the abdomen is shown in Figure 7.

How does it work?

During peritoneal dialysis, sterile dialysate enters the abdomen through the catheter. The waste products, excess substances and fluids in the blood move across the peritoneal membrane into the dialysate. When diffusion (the filtering process) is completed, the used dialysate is allowed to flow out of the abdominal cavity through the catheter, taking with it some of the waste products and excess fluids. It is discarded. Fresh dialysate is sent back in and the treatment is repeated. The number of times the treatment is performed depends on the type of peritoneal dialysis being used.

Are there different types of peritoneal dialysis?

Yes, there are three types:

- continuous ambulatory peritoneal dialysis (CAPD)
- continuous cycling peritoneal dialysis (CCPD)
- intermittent peritoneal dialysis (IPD)

Each type of treatment is based on the same principle, using the peritoneum inside the

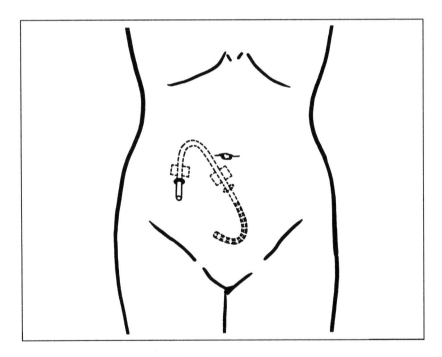

Figure 7.
Peritoneal dialysis catheter

abdominal cavity to remove waste products and excess fluids. However, each treatment is slightly different, as explained further in this chapter.

Continuous ambulatory peritoneal dialysis (CAPD) is performed by you, at home, without the use of a machine. This method of peritoneal dialysis is *continuous*, since the dialysate is in the abdominal cavity 24 hours a day, seven days a week. Fresh dialysate is placed in the abdominal cavity through the catheter four to five times a day, where it sits for four to six hours. This is done by attaching a flexible bag, which holds the dialysate solution, to the catheter using a connecting length of tubing. The container is then raised above the body and gravity pulls the solution into the abdominal cavity. The empty bag is then discarded. During this time, waste products and excess water move from the bloodstream into the dialysate cleansing the blood (see Figure 8).

What is continuous ambulatory peritoneal dialysis (CAPD)?

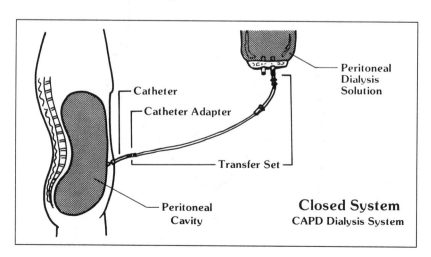

Figure 8.
CAPD process

After a specified time, a new empty bag and a fresh filled bag of dialysate are attached to the catheter. A clamp is opened to allow for drainage into the empty bag. Another clamp is opened to allow refilling of the abdomen with the fresh dialysate. The entire procedure, called an exchange, takes about 35 minutes and is done every four to six hours during the day and eight hours at night to allow for a full night's sleep. Usually, four or five exchanges are required each day.

What is continuous cycling peritoneal dialysis (CCPD)?

Continuous cycling peritoneal dialysis (CCPD), uses a machine called a *cycler* to deliver and drain the dialysate. The procedure is done at home during the night while you sleep. Multiple exchanges take place at night automatically by the cycling machine. In the morning, you make the fourth exchange, leaving dialysate in the abdomen during the day.

What is intermittent peritoneal dialysis (IPD)?

Intermittent peritoneal dialysis (IPD), like CCPD, requires a machine to perform the exchanges. This type of peritoneal dialysis is usually done in a hospital or clinic with the help of trained medical staff. Each treatment requires from 10 to 14 hours and usually occurs three or four times per week.

What are the pros and cons of peritoneal dialysis?

Peritoneal dialysis is the preferred treatment for many people. You may be a better candidate for peritoneal dialysis than hemodialysis if you have poor hemodialysis access routes or heart instability. You also might prefer peritoneal dialysis over hemodialysis because diet and fluid intake is more liberal, and no blood is lost during peritoneal dialysis treatment. Physicians believe that the large fluid gains between hemodialysis treatments place stress on the heart and blood vessels. This is not the case in peritoneal dialysis. Also, there is a reduced need for some medications, particularly antihypertensives.

There are, however, some disadvantages to peritoneal dialysis. There is a possibility of weight gain (fat) caused by the high dextrose, or sugar content, of the dialysate. Older people and diabetics require testing of their blood-sugar level as some of the dextrose in the dialysate is absorbed into the bloodstream and can raise the blood sugar to very high levels. Diabetics, however, may add insulin directly to the dialysis solution.

There are some potential catheter-related problems as well. Infections can occur at the catheter site at the external part of the abdomen. In most cases, these infections can be treated with antibiotics. The most serious problem that can occur is peritonitis or an infection developing inside the abdominal cavity. Peritonitis must be treated with antibiotics, although, in most cases, hospitalization is not necessary. When peritonitis is very severe, however, hospitalization is often advised and you may be dialyzed on a machine continuously with antibiotics in the dialysate, and, sometimes, intravenously as well. The risk of peritonitis can be reduced by using the prescribed sterile technique and close monitoring by your physician.

47

Which type of peritoneal dialysis is best?

The type of peritoneal dialysis you choose depends on your medical condition and personal choice. Your physician and nurses are helpful in this selection.

Are there dietary restrictions for people on peritoneal dialysis?

Yes. Dietary restrictions for people receiving peritoneal dialysis are generally less stringent with respect to protein, salt, potassium and fluids than for those receiving hemodialysis treatment. Patients may, however, need to limit their salt intake, if they have persistent high blood pressure, and to limit phosphorous intake.

Patients may also need to watch calories as there is a tendency to gain weight. A dietitian is helpful in planning the diet.

Where can I get more information about peritoneal dialysis?

Your physician can provide more information. A National Kidney Foundation affiliate can also be contacted for additional literature on peritoneal dialysis.

Treatment For Anemia 5

In the body, blood serves as a liquid transport system. It carries important substances to all cells in the body. It also carries waste materials away from cells.

Blood is made up of fluid (plasma or serum) and contains many different kinds of cells. Red cells, which are called *erythrocytes*, are the most common type. The average person has over 35 trillion erythrocytes. If a person has anemia, they have a reduced number of red blood cells. A doctor can tell how many red blood cells a person has by doing a blood test of the hematocrit or a red blood cell count. The hematocrit tells what percent of the blood is red cells. A normal hematocrit level is between 38% and 48%, but a level of 24 to 30 is satisfactory for a dialysis patient. The doctor may also measure the hemoglobin level. Hemoglobin is the molecule that carries oxygen in red blood cells. A normal hemoglobin level is between 12 grams and 16 grams per deciliter. A normal red blood cell count is between 4.4 and 5.8 million per microliter.

What is anemia?

Hemoglobin in the red blood cells carries oxygen to all parts of the body. The red cells are the oxygen transport system. The body uses oxygen as a fuel or source of energy. When a person is anemic, and does not have enough red blood cells, parts of the body do not get enough oxygen to work properly and

What do red blood cells do?

49

the person may feel tired and out of breath. People with anemia may feel like they have no energy. The hemoglobin in red blood cells also transports carbon dioxide, a waste product from the cells or tissues throughout the body to the lungs where carbon dioxide is excreted.

What are the symptoms of anemia?

Symptoms of anemia include a lack of energy, fatigue, depression and an inability to concentrate or to exercise normally. Shortness of breath, palpitations (rapid or irregular heart beat), impotence (failure to achieve adequate penile erection), dizziness, light-headedness and constantly feeling cold are also symptoms of anemia.

Why do people with kidney disease get anemia?

In the body, a hormone called *erythropoietin* stimulates the bone marrow to control the number of red blood cells. Almost all of the erythropoietin in the body is produced by the kidneys. Erythropoietin travels from the kidneys to the bone marrow, where red blood cells are made. If a person has kidney disease, the kidneys cannot make enough erythropoietin. Without erythropoietin, the bone marrow does not make enough red blood cells to carry oxygen sufficient for the body's needs.

Does dialysis help anemia?

Normally, the kidneys remove fluids and toxins from the blood stream. For people with kidney disease, dialysis does much of this work for the kidneys. However, dialysis cannot replace erythropoietin. Nevertheless, some dialysis patients are not anemic, even without being given erythropoietin.

Dialysis patients may receive blood transfusions if they are anemic. When patients are transfused, they receive red blood cells from a blood donor. They might also receive anabolic male-type (androgenic) hormones, such as decadurabolin. These substances may help raise the hematocrit somewhat.

What methods are available to treat anemia?

Now there is an effective way to treat anemia in people with kidney failure. Scientists have found a way to produce erythropoietin in a laboratory using recombinant DNA technology. This erythropoietin is called *recombinant human erythropoietin,* or *EPO*.

Recombinant human erythropoietin (EPO) is not a drug. It is a hormone, a biologic substance, that is an exact copy of the erythropoietin made by the kidneys. Treatment with EPO is called *replacement therapy*. When you receive EPO treatment, you are just replacing the protein hormone that the kidneys can no longer make. EPO stimulates the bone marrow to produce red blood cells. Once you have enough red blood cells to carry oxygen to all parts of your body you should feel better and have more energy.

What is recombinant human erythropoietin (EPO)?

Patients all over the world have been treated with recombinant human erythropoietin. In almost all of the patients who were treated, their hematocrit and hemoglobin levels rose, which means that they had more red cells in their blood. Once the patients' red cells levels increased, they had more energy, and, in most cases, no longer needed blood transfusions. They could exercise more and lead more active lives.

Is recombinant human erythropoietin effective?

Is recombinant human erythropoietin therapy safe?

EPO treatment is relatively safe and generally very well-tolerated. The doctor checks the blood pressure regularly while you are receiving EPO treatment to make sure that your blood pressure does not go up too high.

The most common side effect of treatment with EPO is an increase in blood pressure. The hematocrit is also monitored, since too high a hematocrit increases the viscosity of the blood, and this also can be harmful; for example, it can increase the risk of clotting an access for hemodialysis.

Why is erythropoietin better than transfusion?

In the past, transfusion was the only effective way to treat anemia in dialysis patients. When you receive a transfusion, you receive red blood cells from a blood donor. However, you can also be at risk of receiving an infection from the blood donor, such as hepatitis (other than Hepatitis B, which is tested for) or even AIDS (if the donor has recent infection and has not yet developed antibodies, which are the basis of the blood test done to screen out the overwhelming majority of infected donors).

Before the advent of human recombinant erythropoietin, anemia in these dialysis patients was treated with androgenic steroid hormones and, if necessary, transfusions of red blood cells.

Both of these treatments had important drawbacks. Androgen (or male) steroids were administered by weekly injection into the muscle. Their mode of action was to stimulate cells in the bone marrow to produce more red blood cells. Unfortunately, androgens had limited effectiveness and, as a side effect, promoted the development of masculine sexual characteristics, such as facial and body hair and deepening of the voice. Blood transfusions are a more effective way of treating anemia. Their usefulness is limited by the danger of transmitting certain viral diseases, such as hepatitis. Furthermore, blood transfusions contain a large amount of iron. Some of the iron is deposited in the liver and other organs. After many units have been given, the iron may cause disease of these organs.

What are the benefits of treatment with recombinant human erythropoietin?

The most important benefit of treatment with recombinant human erythropoietin is an increase in the number of red cells in the blood. Once the number of red blood cells available to carry oxygen to all parts of the body increases, you may not require transfusions, unless you have sudden or substantial bleeding, such as from an ulcer of the stomach or intestine.

Dialysis patients with anemia who have received EPO also experience improved quality of life and sense of well-being. After treatment with EPO, many patients notice an improvement in their ability to work, and their sexual performance, appetite, ability to exercise, social activity, sleep, hair texture and skin color.

Can all people on dialysis with anemia receive recombinant human erythropoietin treatment?

The doctor can say if you should receive recombinant human erythropoietin. The only people who cannot receive EPO are those with uncontrolled high blood pressure or those who may be allergic to the treatment.

53

Will any special tests have to be done during treatment?

Since the doctor wants to make sure that the amount of recombinant human erythropoietin is correct, the hematocrit and hemoglobin levels are measured frequently at the beginning of treatment. Otherwise, no special laboratory tests need be done while you are receiving treatment if you have a normal response to EPO. However, tests for iron, aluminum and vitamins may be done if the response to EPO is slow or inadequate.

Will I need to follow any special procedures while on treatment?

Even though you feel very good while on treatment with EPO, following the diet, dialysis routine and taking the medications the doctor prescribes is very important. Because an increase in blood pressure is a side effect of EPO treatment, you should be especially careful to comply with the doctor's prescription for blood pressure medications.

If you are deficient in iron, you'll probably need to receive iron during treatment. All red blood cells contain iron. Most patients on EPO therapy need extra iron because they are producing red blood cells very quickly in order to keep up with the somewhat rapid destruction and loss of red cells than occurs in normal individuals.

The combination of dialysis, diet medicines and EPO should improve the overall quality of life substantially.

The amount of EPO needed for each patient is different. The doctor determines the starting and maintenance dose.

EPO is given near the end of the hemodialysis treatment. If you are a hemodialysis patient, the doctor or nurse may inject the EPO into the extracorporeal circuit so that you do not have to get another needle-stick. If you are a peritoneal dialysis patient, or dialyze at home, the doctor will instruct you on how you will receive the EPO. Many CAPD patients receive EPO by injection under the skin. This is an effective route of administration for hemodialysis patients as well and may be used in some centers.

How often will I need to take recombinant human erythropoietin?

Kidney Transplantation 6

A kidney transplant is an alternative treatment for kidney failure. In transplantation, a kidney from a living relative or from an unrelated person who has just died is removed and surgically placed into the body.

What is a kidney transplant?

No. Thousands of transplants with high success rates have been performed since the first successful kidney transplant in 1954.

Are kidney transplants experimental?

Children to adults in their sixties or higher may be good candidates for transplantation unless severe medical problems exist.

Who can have a kidney transplant?

A successful transplant provides a quality of life similar to that of a healthy person, unless there are complications of the medications that must be taken to prevent the body from rejecting the kidney. Transplants, however, do not always work, or they may work imperfectly, or there may be complications, such as infections. The decision to have a kidney transplant is based on a patient's medical condition, the ability to adapt to kidney failure, and their personal preference. These factors determine if transplantation is the best choice for the person in their individual situation. Most people feel that life with a transplant is better than life on dialysis.

Is kidney transplantation better than dialysis?

What does success rate in kidney transplantations mean?

Success rate or successful kidney transplantation means that good kidney function is maintained for a sufficient length of time, usually at least one year. Transplants that work well for a year often, but not always, continue to work well for many years.

Where do the donor kidneys come from?

Kidneys for transplantation come from two different sources: a relative (a *living related donor*) or an unrelated person who has died, also called a *cadaver donor*.

Who can be a live donor?

Live donors are typically close family members. Sometimes, more distant relatives or people with whom the patient has a close emotional bond and have a compatible blood type can be donors. Kidneys from living donors usually have a better chance of success.

Who is the best relative to be the donor?

A kidney from an identical twin has the highest success rate. Next is a full brother or sister (especially those 25% of siblings whose tissues are very similar), or a parent-to-child or child-to-parent with the same or compatible blood type. Excellent results can also be achieved nowadays from more distant family members and from non-related donors where there is a close emotional tie, even though the matching between the donor and the recipient may not be close.

What is tissue typing?

Tissue typing is a laboratory test that determines the genetic similarity of the transplant recipient and donor and helps to predict if the transplanted tissue will be accepted or rejected. One of the blood tests is the same as that used in blood transfusions, and is called *blood typing* or *ABO grouping*. Another is HLA typing, which identifies proteins determined by a particular pair of genes within the chromosomes. Though tissue typing is very useful, it is possible to achieve a high degree of success for transplants even when the tissue types appear different. A prediction of success can also be made by what is called sensitivity, which involves comparing the recipient's blood with a random population to determine sensitivity to the various tissue types of the population. A high percentage of sensitivity indicates antibodies in the blood to a high percentage of the population. Before a transplant is performed, the recipient's blood is combined with that of the potential donor to see if there is an unfavorable reaction between them. This test is called a "cross matching."

What does the living kidney donor have to do?

Once the ABO red-blood-cell type has been shown to be compatible, tissue typing is usually performed. A physician must then determine if the living relative is a suitable donor by performing medical and psychological examinations and administering a series of tests. The evaluation involves blood and urine tests, X-rays and an electrocardiogram. If these initial results are normal, a renal arteriogram follows to determine whether or not the blood vessels of the kidney are adequate for transplantation. The results of the evaluation determine if the donor has two normal, healthy kidneys and is, in every other way, a suitable candidate for surgery.

Are there any risks to the related donor?

There are always risks when one undergoes major surgery, but if the living related donor is healthy, the risks are minimal. The donor's

59

remaining kidney takes over the function of the original two kidneys, enlarging in size to handle the increased workload. Many people who were born with only one kidney or had one kidney removed because it was injured or diseased have lived normal lives and have normal lifespans. Limitations to a person with one kidney can include restricting certain physical activities, such as contact sports, in which a severe blow to the area of the one remaining kidney could cause damage.

What happens if I do not have a live donor?

If you do not have a live donor, the kidney may be obtained from a cadaver donor.

What is a cadaver donor kidney?

A cadaver donor kidney is a kidney removed from an unrelated person who has just died. The kidney is briefly stored while tissue typing and cross-matching are done so that a good recipient can be selected. The safe storage time varies, but is usually less than 30 hours (though some kidneys stored for considerably longer have worked well).

How will I know whose kidney I receive?

In the case of a cadaver donor kidney, the general policy in the United States is not to disclose the name of the donor to the recipient and not to give the name of the recipient to the donor's family.

How long will I have to wait for a cadaver kidney?

The waiting period for a cadaver kidney transplant depends upon the availability of a matching cadaver donor. Sometimes, the wait can be a year or longer, and other times can be much less. Your physician can discuss the waiting time.

The Uniform Anatomical Gift Act makes available on a national basis the Uniform Donor Card (a donor sticker is used in some states), a wallet-sized legal document signed by the carrier and stating the carrier's desire to donate any or all parts of their body at the time of death. Any person of sound mind, 18 years of age or older, can sign this card. Whether or not a donor card is present on the deceased at the time of death, the next of kin makes the final decision regarding the kidneys or other organs of the deceased relative. Federal regulations require hospitals to ask family members when a relative dies to consider donating the family member's kidneys and other organs or tissues. This is called "routine inquiry" or "required request."

Where do the cadaver kidneys come from?

Cadaver kidneys constitute almost 70 percent of the kidneys used in transplantation worldwide. The National Kidney Foundation affiliate can provide more information on donating kidneys and also a donor card for anyone who wishes one.

You should speak with your physician about your interest in transplantation, and obtain further information about the success of transplantation, types of donors and the complications of transplantation. You should also seek a willing donor among your relatives, and discuss the type of donor, living related or cadaver you would like with your family and physician. You can assure family members that a physician will not accept a kidney from a living donor if they believe that there is significant risk to that donor.

How do I get a kidney?

61

If you are to receive a living donor kidney, the following will be arranged and completed prior to transplant:

- tissue typing from both yourself and the potential donor
- a full donor workup or medical evaluation
- periodic physical examinations by the local nephrologist or transplant center
- blood tests and X-rays (and possibly other tests)

If you are to receive a transplant from a cadaver, the following will be completed before your name is placed on a waiting list:

- you are tissue-typed and the results placed in a computer with other names on the waiting list
- a tube of blood serum must be sent regularly from the dialysis center to the tissue-typing laboratory for sensitivity screening
- periodic physical examinations, X-rays and blood tests are ordered

Also, the hospital or dialysis center must be assured of your whereabouts by receiving the telephone numbers and addresses so that you can be reached if a kidney becomes available. (Sometimes telepagers are used.)

What happens if a cadaver kidney becomes available?

You are notified when a potential kidney is available. Once notified, you should stay close to a phone to receive information on the time of hospital admission. Arrangements for traveling to the hospital should be made and you will probably be told not to eat or drink anything in preparation for surgery. You may need to be dialyzed before the surgery depending upon when you were last dialyzed, your blood chemistries and your general medical condition.

The kidney to be transplanted is placed in the pelvic area, just under the abdominal muscles, rather than in the usual location in the flank (back). The locations of the natural kidneys and a transplanted kidney are shown in Figure 9. The artery that carries blood to the kidney and the vein that removes blood from it are surgically connected with two blood vessels already existing in the pelvis. The ureter, or tube, that carries urine from the kidney is then connected to the bladder. The transplant operation takes about three hours.

What happens in the transplant operation?

Surgical risks as a person with kidney failure are greater than those for people with normal kidney function. However, the survival rate from transplant surgery is greater than 95 percent.

Are there risks in the transplant operation?

Nephrectomy is the removal of a kidney. In a few cases, kidneys may have to be surgically removed some time before the transplant in an operation called *bilateral nephrectomy*. The most common reason for recommending a nephrectomy is the presence of repeated infection in the kidneys or extremely severe hypertension.

What is a nephrectomy?

In the same way that the body fights bacteria and viruses that cause illness, it also resists the presence of a foreign substance or cells or tissues from an outside source. This rejection process can result in the body's resistance to

What does rejection mean?

63

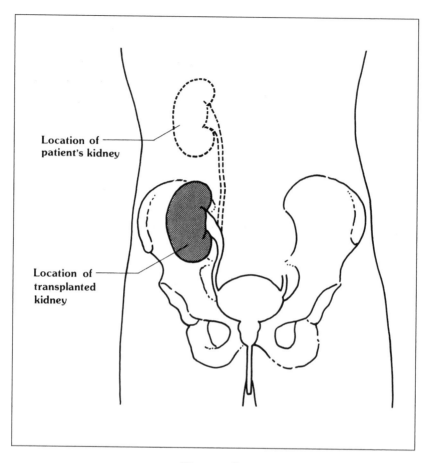

Figure 9.
Location of kidney before and after transplant

kidney tissue transplanted from another human being. Many people who receive a kidney transplant experience some degree of rejection. A period of rejection does not necessarily mean that they will lose the kidney. There are two general types of rejection: acute and chronic.

Acute rejection is the most common form of rejection and is sometimes difficult to diagnose. Prompt treatment can reverse the rejection in most cases. Acute rejection may be detected by laboratory tests before symptoms appear. With a sudden onset of acute rejection, the patient may have fever, generalized aching, sudden weight gain, a decrease in the amount of urine produced and tenderness over the area of the transplanted kidney.

What is the difference between acute and chronic rejection?

Acute rejection also can occur without any obvious symptoms. Although acute rejection is most frequent during the first three months after transplantation, it may occur after months or even years. Antirejection therapy with certain medications is continued indefinitely to combat the acute rejection, and ongoing laboratory studies of kidney function are performed to detect worsening of kidney function, which may occur without symptoms. If acute rejection occurs, treatment can include ongoing visits to a physician, and, in some cases in which acute rejection is severe, hospitalization.

Chronic rejection is the continuous tendency of the body to reject the kidney. Chronic rejection does not occur in everyone, but is more likely to occur if the patient has had several episodes of acute rejection. There are usually few signs of chronic rejection, though there may be a tendency toward swelling (or edema) and weight gain. Chronic rejection is usually diagnosed by repeated laboratory tests and can often be slowed, with careful medical treatment, to allow ongoing function of the transplanted kidney. If the patient experiences chronic rejection, they will need frequent physician visits and possibly adjustment in medications as well as dietary restrictions.

Yet another form of rejection is *hyperacute rejection*. This rare form of rejection can occur within minutes or hours after transplantation and can cause irreversible destruction of the transplanted kidney. Fortunately, this type of rejection is not very common.

How long does it take to recover after transplant surgery?

The recovery period varies with each individual and depends upon the severity of the rejection threat the amount of medication needed, how quickly the transplanted kidney functions, how well you tolerate the antirejection medication, and complications that can occur with any operative procedure. It could take a few weeks to a month or even longer.

What are the chances of a transplant being a success?

Your success rate depends on whether the kidney comes from a living relative or cadaver donor. The success rate, or the percentage of kidney transplants that achieve and maintain good function, is usually better when the kidney comes from a living relative. Although individual transplant programs may have varied results, most programs achieve an overall success rate of 85 percent or higher.

How long will a transplant last?

Many people who received transplants more than 20 years ago still have functioning kidneys, though many kidney transplants do not last that long. Many people return for a second transplant after losing their first. The length of time you keep the transplanted kidney depends on your individual situation.

If the body totally rejects the transplanted kidney in the first several months, or if it fails to function, the transplanted kidney may need to be surgically removed from the body. A patient then returns to dialysis, and, if they choose, wait for another available kidney. Late failure of the transplant may not require its removal.

What happens if the transplant is rejected or fails to work?

Yes, unless you receive a kidney from an identical twin. You are required to take medications or anti-rejection drugs, known as immunosuppressants, as long as the transplanted kidney is functioning.

Will I need to take medications after the transplant?

The purpose of treatment with immunosuppressant drugs is to alter the body's defense mechanism in its response toward the transplanted kidney. Current forms of immunosuppressants used are prednisone, azathioprine, cyclosporine, FK506, antilymphocyte globulin and OKT3. Immunosuppressant drugs help combat the body's rejection of the transplanted kidney.

What are immunosuppressant drugs and why are they important?

Yes. As with many drugs, there are side effects to immunosuppressants. One effect, which all immunosuppressant drugs can produce, is infection. The drugs not only alter the body's immune system in its response toward the transplanted kidney, but also alter the proper response toward invading microorganisms, such as bacteria, viruses and fungi. A patient is more susceptible to infections, which sometimes can be serious, even fatal. Signs of infection can include chills, fever, reddened areas, tenderness, swelling, cough and

Are there side effects to immunosuppressant drugs?

67

discharges. Any of these should be reported to a physician. Each drug, whether it is prednisone, azathioprine, cyclosporine, antilymphocyte globulin or Orthoclone OKT3, also can produce specific side effects.

The effects of prednisone are often influenced by the dosage given. It can be administered the day prior to or on the day of transplantation in high dosages according to body weight. Over a period of four to six months, the dosage may be reduced to what is called a maintenance or minimal dose. Thereafter, a patient must take this dosage of prednisone as long as the kidney is working. If rejection occurs, the dosage may be increased. During the high dose period of prednisone, the following side effects may occur:

- susceptibility to infection
- salt accumulation in the body resulting in fluid retention
- irritation of the gastrointestinal tract causing heartburn
- hormonal changes, such as thinning of the hair, acne, facial hair growth and mood swings
- bone involvement causing joint pain
- delay in wound healing
- redistribution of fat deposited in cheeks, abdomen and back
- possible development of diabetes, cataracts or hypertension

Many of these side effects are, to a large part, reversible as the dosage of prednisone is lowered.

Azathioprine, which is used in conjunction with prednisone and sometimes with cyclosporine, is usually started on the day of transplantation. The dosage of azathioprine usually remains roughly the same throughout the life of the kidney. Azathioprine can reduce the production of white blood cells in the bone marrow, which can increase susceptibility to infection. When the white cell count is too low, the azathioprine dosage may be reduced or discontinued until the white cell count returns to a safe level. Azathioprine may also cause anemia, a reduction of the number of red cells in the blood because of decreased production.

The most important recent development in organ transplantation is the introduction of cyclosporine as an alternative immunosuppressant medication. Cyclosporine has had a major impact on the success rates of kidney transplants and has been partially responsible for the increased popularity of transplantation among people with kidney failure. This immunosuppressant is usually given intravenously, usually for the first several days, and, thereafter, is given orally. It may be started on the day of the transplant or a few days later. Cyclosporine can interfere with the function of the transplant and, for this reason, the concentration of this drug in the blood must be checked frequently and modifications made in the dosage, if necessary.

Antilymphocyte globulin (ALG), antithymocyte globulin (ATG) and the monoclonal antibody OKT3 are three powerful drugs usually given to treat severe rejection that has not responded to treatment with high doses of prednisone. Some transplant centers may use one of these drugs to prevent rejection.

69

If I have had a kidney transplant, will I need a special diet? In most cases, you may eat and drink whatever you desire. Sometimes, you may need to follow a low-sodium diet because of the medications required for rejection and the ability to cause fluid retention in your body tissue. Also, sodium restriction is required if you have high blood pressure. You may need to be careful about calories because of a tendency to gain weight.

What are the advantages of kidney transplantation over dialysis? The advantages of kidney transplantation over dialysis may include better health, better quality of life, absence of need for frequent dialysis treatments and reduced medical costs after the first year. A woman of childbearing age may be able to have children and a man may have a better chance of fathering children.

What are the disadvantages of a kidney transplant? The disadvantages of kidney transplantation may include the pain and discomfort of surgery; risk of rejection; the need for frequent physician visits and possible hospitalization as a result of the anti-rejection drugs; the inability to fight off infections, which may occasionally be life threatening; some permanent conditions caused by drugs, including eye cataracts, arthritis and even cancer (most commonly, a treatable form of skin cancer); the cost of the anti-rejection drugs; and ongoing anxiety caused by the fear of losing the transplanted kidney's function and returning to another form of dialysis.

The average kidney transplant without complications in the United States costs approximately $34,000. This cost covers the transplant surgeon's fee, hospitalization, tests, laboratory fees, medication, anesthesiologist, operating room, nursing care and costs related to organ donation for both living related and deceased donors. Medicare benefits, regardless of age, cover most of these costs. Medicare coverage of the anti-rejection drugs, however, occurs for only the first year after transplant. Some state Medicaid programs and private insurance companies cover costs not covered by Medicare. The provisions of the Omnibus Budget Reconciliation Act of 1993 (OBRA '93) extend the period for immunosuppressant drug therapy from one year to three based on the following timetable:

How much does kidney transplantation cost?

- For patients furnished drugs before 1995, the coverage remains for 12 months after the date of transplant
- Medication furnished during 1995 is covered for 18 months
- During 1996, coverage extends to a full two years
- Those receiving immunosuppressants during 1997 will receive 30 months of coverage
- For any year after 1997, benefits remain in place for a full three years. OBRA '93 takes effect on January 1, 1995

Diet and Medication

The information on diet in this chapter refers mainly to the needs of people on hemodialysis. People on peritoneal dialysis or who have kidney transplants require fewer dietary adjustments.

Healthy kidneys regulate the levels of most substances in the body, including blood levels of sodium, potassium bicarbonate, calcium, phosphorus, fluid and protein waste products. The kidneys clear the blood of excess amounts of these substances to keep the body in balance. When the kidneys are not functioning properly, these substances can build up to dangerous levels in the blood and may cause you to have symptoms of uremia, which includes a loss of appetite, nausea, vomiting, itching, twitching and less often a wide variety of other symptoms. Dialysis removes some, but not all, of these waste products. For this reason, diet control is an important part of managing kidney disease.

Why must I change my diet?

No. Each person is different. The type of diet that a person needs depends on age, weight, the percentage of kidney function they have remaining, the effectiveness of dialysis treatment to rid their body of excess waste products and fluids and whether or not they have other medical complications.

Do all people with kidney disease require the same dietary adjustments?

What are the most common dietary adjustments? The most common dietary changes include adjusting the intake of the following nutrients in the diet: protein, calories, sodium, potassium, phosphorus, water and other fluids.

Why is protein important? Protein supplies the body with the building blocks needed for maintenance, growth and repair of body tissues, as well as to assure that a person feels well and can fight off disease. The body can use protein, as well as carbohydrates or fat, to provide energy, since every living cell in the body requires a source of energy. This energy is provided by three of the nutrients in the foods a person eats. These are carbohydrates (starches, sugars and fruits), fats (vegetable oil, margarine and butter), and protein (meat, poultry, eggs, and fish). The body's energy needs are very important. If carbohydrates and fats are not available, the body uses protein for energy, and if it is used for energy, it is not available to build tissue. Furthermore, if there are insufficient calories in the diet, the body may digest its own tissues that are made up of protein.

Why is protein regulated in the diet? When protein is metabolized, it produces waste products, one of which is called *urea*. When the kidneys are not functioning, urea cannot be eliminated from the body and can build up in the blood. A test that can determine the amount of urea present in the blood is called *blood urea nitrogen (BUN)*. The BUN can be high if too much protein is eaten, the wrong kind of protein is eaten and if not enough calories are eaten. High levels of BUN are associated with nausea, vomiting and loss of appetite. The protein intake is limited to prevent the BUN from becoming too high. The diet requires you to eat foods with good quality protein because these provide the essential building blocks for body tissues. These proteins include meats, fish, poultry, eggs, milk and cheeses. The BUN can become low if you do not eat enough protein. Too little protein can cause the muscle tissues to break down and lead to malnutrition, causing additional medical problems, including decreased resistance to infection. Therefore, it is important that you follow a protein prescription to assure that your body is getting the protein it needs and that the amount of waste products are kept within acceptable ranges.

What is the difference between good quality protein and poor quality protein?

Good quality protein contains the essential building blocks known as amino acids needed to build and repair body tissues. Foods that contain good quality or high-biological-value protein are those from animal sources and are found in eggs, meat, poultry and fish. Foods that contain poor quality protein or low-biological-value protein are those from plant sources and cannot be used alone to build and repair body tissues. Poor-quality protein can be found in breads, cereals, pastas and vegetables. At least 50 percent of necessary protein should come from foods with good quality protein.

Are calories important?

A calorie is a measurement of the energy value of food. A well-balanced diet provides the protein one needs for growth of tissues and blood cells and enough calories to meet the body's energy needs. When enough calories

75

are present in the diet, the body does not rely on protein as an energy source and the valuable proteins are allowed to perform the other important functions. The body stores energy as fat when you consume more calories than your body needs; it can also use stored fat for energy when you consume fewer calories than it needs. Calorie requirements depend on age, activity level, weight, sex, type of treatment and other medical problems that may exist. The diet a dietitian gives you will include a sufficient caloric intake to meet your individual needs and activity level.

What is potassium and why is it important? Potassium is a mineral needed for normal function of nerves and muscles. Since the heart is a large muscle, the amount of potassium in the blood affects the beating of the heart. When kidney function is normal, excess potassium is excreted in the urine. When the kidneys are not functioning properly, potassium builds up in the blood until it is removed by dialysis. If this level of potassium in the blood becomes too high, it can cause muscle weakness and may affect the heartbeat. Just as high blood potassium level can be dangerous, so can a low blood potassium level by causing the heart to beat irregularly.

Which foods contain a lot of potassium? Some of the foods rich in potassium include potatoes, dark green leafy vegetables, citrus fruits, bananas, tomatoes, avocados, winter squash, dried beans and peas and nuts. A physician and dietitian will give you a diet with the appropriate potassium content.

Learning the potassium content of various foods is important.

Yes. Some of the potassium from certain foods, such as potatoes and other vegetables, can be removed by peeling and slicing these foods very thinly and soaking them in a large amount of water for 24 hours. This can reduce the potassium content up to one half. This is sometimes referred to as *dialyzing* or *leaching* vegetables. Once the soaking is completed, the water should be discarded and not re-used.

Can potassium be removed from food?

Usually, no obvious warning signs appear when a body is taking in too much potassium. Excess potassium or hyperkalemia can be very serious and can cause muscle weakness and an irregular heartbeat, and can even cause the heart to stop beating. You can prevent high levels of potassium in your blood by carefully following your prescribed diet. The serum potassium is tested periodically to assure that your blood level is within the acceptable range (serum is the liquid portion of the blood). It is also possible to have a low blood potassium level or hypokalemia, which can sometimes cause you to feel weak. A low potassium level is treated by increasing the dietary intake of potassium with guidance provided by a dietitian. Your physician may also prescribe supplemental potassium medication if your body's potassium is seriously depleted, as may happen if you develop diarrhea.

What happens if I eat too much potassium or too little?

What is sodium?

Sodium is an important mineral found in almost all foods. It is found in the body's tissues and helps to regulate fluid content and blood pressure.

Are sodium and salt the same thing?

Not exactly. Salt does contain sodium, but it also contains chloride. All foods contain some sodium, even if they do not all have added salt.

Is sodium restriction a part of the diet?

Yes. If you have hypertension or edema (excessive fluid in the body), you must restrict sodium intake. In most cases, when the kidneys are not functioning, sodium cannot be excreted. The excess sodium can cause the accumulation of excess body fluids. For this reason, sodium is usually moderately to strictly controlled in your diet. Excess sodium can cause fluid to build up in your body tissue (edema), which can place an extra strain on your heart and may cause high blood pressure.

What foods contain a lot of sodium?

The most common source of sodium in the diet is table salt. Foods high in sodium content include cured, processed and smoked meats, such as ham, bacon, sausage and cold cuts; foods that are salty to the taste, such as potato chips, pretzels, corn chips, salted nuts and pickles; certain condiments, such as prepared mustard, relishes, catsup, seasonings, monosodium glutamate, steak and meat sauces, soy sauce and meat tenderizers; and most processed and canned foods and packaged entrees. Becoming familiar with the sodium content of the different foods is important. Sometimes, canned and packaged foods include a label with the sodium content.

If you eat foods high in sodium, the excess level of sodium in your body can cause symptoms, such as:

- sudden weight gain
- puffiness or swelling of your face, feet, ankles, legs and sometimes your arms and abdomen
- difficulty in breathing because of extra fluid loads on the heart and in the lungs
- a feeling of being bloated or uncomfortable

Excess sodium can also cause high blood pressure, which is not always obvious. You can control the sodium level in your body by following a prescribed dietary plan.

What happens if I eat too much sodium?

No, because the main ingredient of most salt substitutes is potassium. Salt substitutes should never be used unless you check with your dietitian or physician. Some salt substitutes do not have potassium.

Can I use salt substitutes?

Yes. Calcium is the most abundant element in the body; 95 percent of your body's calcium is located in your bones and teeth. Phosphorus is the second most abundant element in the body, and a large percentage of your body's phosphorus is combined with the calcium in your bone structure. A lesser amount of phosphorus is found in the soft tissues and fluids of your body. Both calcium and phosphorus are needed to form bones. The body cannot make use of calcium unless active Vitamin D is present. Because nonfunctioning kidneys cannot activate Vitamin D, calcium from the food you eat cannot be absorbed well. As a result, your blood level of calcium can drop.

Are calcium and phosphorus important in my diet?

79

Phosphorus can build up in your blood when your kidneys are not functioning, which can also cause a decrease in the level of blood calcium. When calcium levels fall, the parathyroid glands secrete the parathyroid hormone, which causes calcium to be released from the bones and sent back into the bloodstream. This release of calcium from your bones can cause them to become brittle or weak, and if this process continues unchecked your bones can break. A physician monitors this delicate relationship between calcium and phosphorus in your body and may prescribe a calcium supplement. You should restrict foods high in phosphorus from your diet. Phosphate binders (usually calcium salts) may also be prescribed to prevent the phosphorus in your food from being absorbed into your body.

Why must I restrict my intake of phosphorus?

Because high levels of phosphorus in your blood can help to rob bones of needed calcium, restricting phosphorus in your diet is important. In addition, high levels of phosphorus may combine with calcium and deposit in the soft tissues, such as your blood vessels, lungs and skin, which may contribute to itching, joint pains and eye irritation.

What foods are high in phosphorus?

Foods high in phosphorus include milk and other dairy products, beans, nuts, cola drinks, whole grain cereals and other foods. A dietitian provides you with a list of foods high in phosphorus.

Yes. Properly functioning kidneys prevent fluid in your body from building up by removing the excess fluid through urine. When your kidneys are not functioning, fluid accumulates in your tissues and bloodstream and may place a strain on your heart as well as cause high blood pressure. Fluid can also collect in your lungs, making it hard to breathe.

Is it important to control fluid intake?

A physician may or may not put you on fluid restriction. If your physician does put you on fluid restriction, you will have to determine how much fluid you can have in a day. A dietitian can also help you plan your fluid intake.

How much fluid can I have each day?

It is important for you to learn how to measure the amount of fluid you can drink. Fluids can be measured in cubic centimeters, ounces, tablespoons or cups:

1 tablespoon = 1/2 fluid ounce = 15 cc.
2 tablespoons = 1 fluid ounce = 30 cc.
1/4 cup = 2 ounces = 60 cc.
1/2 cup = 4 ounces = 120 cc.
1 cup = 8 ounces = 240 cc.
4 cups = 960 cc. = approx. 1 liter

In measuring the amount of fluid taken in, the patient should be aware that even solid foods contain substantial quantities of fluid. Any food that is liquid at room temperature, such as ice cream, popsicles or Jello, must be counted as fluid. Crushed ice is a good way to satisfy thirst and keep fluid intake down, but ice must also be counted in fluid intake. Weighing oneself at the same time each day is a good way to watch how well one is doing in fluid intake. Gaining up to a pound a day between dialysis treatments is usually considered a reasonable weight gain. As a general rule, one pint (16 ounces) of extra fluid equals approximately a one pound weight gain. A dietitian can give you more information on what foods are high in fluids as well as give tips on what to do when you are thirsty (i.e., on how to satisfy thirst without excessive fluid intake).

Is it possible to not get enough fluid?

Occasionally, people with kidney failure do not take in enough fluid. If this happens, they may experience the symptoms of dehydration, including lightheadedness, muscle cramps and feeling faint, weak and nauseated. Low blood pressure (hypotension) can occur until fluid balance is restored.

Can I drink alcoholic beverages?

In most cases, alcoholic beverages are permitted for people with kidney failure. Any alcoholic beverages consumed must be included in the fluid allowance. You should also get prior authorization from your physician before drinking alcoholic beverages.

What does dry weight mean?

The term dry weight is often used by physicians and other professional staff. Dry weight is what people weigh when all excess fluid has been removed from their bodies by dialysis treatment.

Should I take vitamins to supplement a restricted diet?

A controlled diet might limit your vitamin intake, and dialysis treatments can remove some vitamins from your body. Therefore, a physician prescribes supplementary vitamins and certain minerals. Any additional vitamins should be taken under the advice of a physician.

Yes. You must make some adjustments while receiving peritoneal dialysis treatments. For most people, however, there are fewer dietary changes, and less, if any, fluid restriction, required for peritoneal dialysis than for hemodialysis.

Will I need to make dietary adjustments on peritoneal dialysis?

Yes. Some dietary changes are necessary if you receive a kidney transplant. You will find, however, the diet with a transplant is very similar to the diet before kidney failure.

Will I need to change my diet if I receive a transplant?

You will probably follow a diabetic diet with a few changes while on hemodialysis. You may need to substitute some fat for protein to maintain caloric intake while reducing the protein level. A physician will monitor your blood sugar level closely. If you are receiving peritoneal dialysis, the level of protein in your diet may be increased and the carbohydrates absorbed from the dialysate are considered in your total caloric intake. This may require your insulin to be adjusted. Your physician and dietitian will help you plan a diet that meets your individual needs while receiving dialysis treatment.

What if I am diabetic?

A dietitian at the dialysis unit is a valuable resource person to help with your dietary plan. This person can help identify foods that should be restricted in your diet as well as those that should be increased in your dietary intake. A dietitian can also help to put these foods into the form of a daily menu.

Where can I go to find help in planning my menu?

Familiarizing yourself with foods and their contents is important. To help get you started, a table of selected foods and their contents is included in Appendix B.

Can I still eat in restaurants?

Yes. Once you understand your diet, you will know what foods are safe to order from the menu. You will probably have to limit or avoid foods that are high in sodium and potassium. When you eat in a restaurant, it is a good idea to avoid stews, casseroles and cream sauces, because these menu items could include hidden ingredients that you will want to avoid. You should not hesitate to request your food be prepared without salt. Most restaurants are very willing to cooperate with special dietary needs.

Are there special cookbooks available?

Yes. More and more cookbooks are being written and published for people with kidney failure. A list of special cookbooks can be found in Appendix C. A simple, but important, rule to follow before you use any recipes is to discuss them with your dietitian. This way, you will know that they comply with any special dietary needs.

What do I need to know about measurements?

The meal plans given to you by dietitians may include dietary restrictions, suggested menus, recipes and other dietary information that includes various weights and measurements. You may run across liquid measurements in the form of milliliters (ml) and dry measurements in the form of grams (gm). To help you understand some of the measurements, a table of weights and measurements is included in Appendix D.

What medications will I need?

In addition to dietary regulations, a physician will require you to take certain prescribed medications. The medications taken serve a variety of purposes, including lowering your blood pressure, increasing your calcium level in your blood, preventing phosphate from being absorbed in your body and increasing production of red blood cells. A list of some of the most common types of drugs, their brand names and their purposes has been included in Appendix E. This list includes only some of the most common drugs used to deal with conditions related to kidney failure. Your physician may prescribe other drugs not mentioned.

What are phosphate binders?

Phosphate (phosphorus) binders, or antacids, are used to prevent the absorption of phosphorus by binding it up in the intestines. Phosphate is present in most foods, and for this reason, the antacids should be taken just before or while eating, or immediately after a meal. Once the phosphorus is bound to the antacid, it passes out of the body in the stool. A physician will ask a patient not to take any other medications at the time they take the antacid, because they, too, may be bound. Besides binding phosphorus, antacids also bind other drugs. The type of antacid taken is important and must be taken with a physician's approval. Some antacids contain ingredients that may be harmful. Many contain magnesium, which is usually not allowed, but may occasionally be prescribed.

What do analgesics do?

Analgesics are medications that relieve pain. Some analgesics also reduce fever. Tylenol is an example of an analgesic, as is aspirin. A patient is instructed, however, never to take aspirin for any reason unless ordered by a physician. Aspirin often causes bleeding in the stomach and can alter clotting time.

Will I need antibiotics?

An antibiotic is a medication that either stops the growth of bacteria or kills bacteria. You may, on occasion, have infections and require antibiotics. They can be given in pill form or by injections, depending on the antibiotic and the severity of the infection.

What are calcium supplements?

Calcium tablets increase the amount of calcium in the blood and body and also act as antacids and as phosphate binders. They are taken orally.

Will I need any medications for the heart?

A physician may prescribe blood pressure medications to lower your blood pressure. Another type of medication sometimes used to make your heartbeat stronger, slower, and more regular is a heart stimulant called digitalis or Digoxin.

What drugs promote red blood cell production?

Because folic acid is removed from the blood during dialysis treatment and is necessary for normal red blood cell production, it must be replaced to avoid anemia. You may be asked to take a folic acid tablet every day. Besides folic acid, you may need iron medications to maintain a normal blood iron level and thereby provide an adequate amount of iron for normal red blood cell production. Occasionally patients will be given male hormone (androgen) shots or pills to stimulate their body to make more red blood cells. Recombinant human erythropoietin (EPO) is now available and is used for most people on dialysis. This promotes red blood cell production, and more than any other medication, is responsible for correcting the anemia of kidney (renal) failure and avoiding the need for transfusions.

Will I need laxatives?

Stool softeners and dietary or medicinal fiber act to soften the stool. Some laxatives stimulate the bowel to be more active. A physician may recommend that you take a stool softener or certain laxatives, since phosphate builders may cause constipation.

What is Vitamin D and what does it do?

Vitamin D, or calcitriol (the active form of Vitamin D), causes the body to absorb calcium from food and place it in the bones. Vitamin D and calcitriol come in capsules, which are taken orally. Depending on a persons' blood calcium level, a physician may or may not prescribe this drug. There are several forms of Vitamin D used to treat people on dialysis. The most common one is calcitriol by mouth or by vein, but a physician may recommend one of the other forms.

Will I need vitamin supplements?

Most people with kidney failure require vitamin supplements. Supplements are used to replace any vitamins removed during dialysis or not being sufficiently provided by their diet. There are many brands of vitamins, but most contain folic acid, Vitamin C and the Vitamin B complex. These are the ones most dializable. Vitamin supplements should be taken with a physician's guidance. Multivitamins containing large amounts of vitamin A, E or C should be avoided.

Adjustment and Rehabilitation   8

This question is difficult to answer because each person reacts differently to their kidney failure and treatment. Learning to live with dialysis may be a minor adjustment or it may demand a major change in lifestyle or even philosophy. Any important change in your life requires altering habits, priorities, schedules and outlook. Each person receiving treatment for kidney failure is an individual, and that individuality remains after kidney function is lost.

How will having kidney failure change my life?

Most people with chronic illness experience some degree of depression and anxiety. Since kidney failure and treatment is a chronic condition, *not* a terminal one, you may also experience feelings of sorrow, grief, confusion, fear and even anger. These feelings are normal and many people going through what you are will also have these feelings. As you become familiar and comfortable with treatment, your ability to deal with these feelings and concerns, and kidney failure and treatment will become a part of your lifestyle.

Should I expect some emotional problems as a result of kidney failure?

Most people experience depression at some point in their lives. Depression, or feelings of sadness, unhappiness and despair, can occur with stress, loss and illness. Depression can cause a loss of appetite, decreased interest in sex and difficulty in sleeping. One way to deal

Is depression normal?

with depression is to talk about it; usually, talking about it helps people to understand why they are depressed. They should communicate with family and friends and talk with their social worker. In many cases, understanding the depression helps to deal with the problem causing it.

What is anxiety? Anxiety is uneasiness or apprehension concerning an anticipated event or problem. If a person is anxious, they may have *excessive* perspiration, rapid pulse and heart rate, tiredness, irritability or agitation. Very often, the cause of anxiety cannot be determined. Many people who have a chronic illness experience some degree of anxiety. Like depression, the best way to deal with anxiety is to talk it through with someone—a friend, a family member, a minister, the social worker or other mental health professional.

How do I cope? There is no single way of coping with kidney failure and treatment. Because each person has a different experience with, and attitude toward, dialysis, you must find your own individual way of coping. There are, however, several suggestions that other people with kidney failure have made to ease adjustment to chronic illness and treatment, including education about kidney failure and treatment, physical fitness, communication in maintaining important personal relationships and motivation to complete projects and goals.

Education or information about kidney failure and selected treatment is very important. Knowledge of what is happening inside your body, the reaction to dialysis, why medication is needed and why certain foods and fluids must be restricted is crucial to your overall understanding of what is happening. The feeling of helplessness and dependency on the medical staff can be reduced by knowing and understanding kidney failure and treatment. Putting this knowledge to use will help you to feel better and can give you a sense of being in control of your own life. Fears and anxieties can be the result of lack of information; the unknown, which we all fear, can become known through education.

Physical fitness should be important to everyone with or without kidney failure. Mild and regular exercise can help rebuild strength, help insomnia and anemia and strengthen bones and muscles. A physical fitness and exercise program developed with the help of a physician can give you a feeling of accomplishment and overall well-being.

Communication is one way to maintain important personal relationships. Talking things through with your partner, family members and friends is very important in maintaining relationships. Sharing feelings, concerns, fear and anger with others not only helps you feel better, it will also help your family and friends in understanding and accepting what is going on inside. Closing out those people important to you can hurt the relationship by making them feel no longer needed or wanted. Ongoing communication, like education, may help you to become aware of your feelings. Once you are aware of your own feelings, you can begin to accept kidney failure as an unfortunate, but challenging, part of life, and you can go on living.

Motivation, setting personal goals, completing projects and continuing to lead life as close as possible to the way you did before kidney failure is very important. Continuing enjoyable activities, being with loved ones and continuing to plan your life should not change with kidney failure. Most people's feelings of self-esteem or self-worth depend on what they do and accomplish. Although kidney failure and treatment can change some external aspects of your life, your essential worth and value to yourself and others can and should remain unchanged.

Will my mental attitude affect my physical health?

Your emotional state can affect your physical health and, in the case of kidney failure, can affect medical treatment and progress. If your emotional state or mental attitude is positive, you will most likely do well on dialysis. If, however, you are having a difficult time adjusting, or had problems prior to the kidney failure, you may not do as well on dialysis as someone with a positive mental outlook.

Will my illness affect my marriage and family?

Family members face many of the emotional stresses and problems that you do, including depression, anxiety, concern for life expectancy, concern about finances, difficulty in expressing honest feelings and concern over sexual competence. In some cases, discussion groups, in which family members express their concerns and provide mutual emotional support, can help your family to adapt to your illness. The social worker can provide more information.

In some cases, uremia, the building up of waste products in the bloodstream between dialysis treatments, can affect thinking. Sometimes, a person may experience difficulty in remembering things, inability to concentrate and confusion. On rare occasions, they may lose contact with reality or experience hallucinations. Experiencing things, like seeing, hearing, tasting, feeling or smelling things that do not exist, can be very frightening. If this happens, it is important for you to tell your physician. Some people who experience hallucinations do not tell anyone for fear that they are losing their minds, when in reality, the hallucinations can be caused by inadequate dialysis treatments, the need for medications or by fever and infection (delirium).

Can kidney failure affect my thinking?

Sometimes, your desire for sexual activity, or sexual appetite, changes with chronic illness. The ability to enjoy sex, on the part of the male or female, depends on you as an individual. Impotence, or the inability of a male to have an erection or to maintain an erection, can occur. Problems with ejaculation are also a possibility. However, your ability to participate in sexual activity and to enjoy sex is still possible. If you find your sex life changing, talk to your physician or social worker, because these problems may be treatable. Very often, the stress and anxiety related to kidney failure and treatment can affect your sexual appetite and ability to enjoy sex.

Can I still enjoy sex?

Where can I read about other people who are going through what I am?

Several magazines have been published that include articles about kidney treatment and adjustment. Magazines that deal with current issues related to kidney failure, dialysis and transplantation are:

Renalife
The AAKP Bulletin
Write to: AAKP, 111 South Parker Street, Suite 405, Tampa, FL 33606.

FOR PATIENTS ONLY
Write to: Contemporary Dialysis, Inc., 6300 Variel Avenue, Suite 1, Woodland Hills, CA 91364.

Family Focus
Write to: National Kidney Foundation, 30 East 33rd St., 11th floor, New York, NY 10016.

PATIENT ADVISORY NEWS
Write to: Network Council, #18 6255 Sunset Blvd., Suite 2211, Hollywood, CA 90028.

How can I meet and talk with other people who have kidney failure?

The American Association of Kidney Patients (AAKP) is an organization of patients for patients. The purpose of AAKP is to promote the welfare of kidney patients through education and advocacy. Although the national office is located in Florida, there are local chapters in many parts of the United States. These chapters offer educational meetings and social activities that bring patients and families together. For more information on the AAKP and the closest chapter, contact AAKP at (800) 749-2257.

Some National Kidney Foundation affiliates also offer educational meetings for people with kidney failure. For more information on the National Kidney Foundation meetings, contact the local National Kidney Foundation affiliate.

Where can I find help?

If you or your family need help to adjust and cope with kidney failure, you should talk to a social worker. A social worker is a valuable resource person and can help you and your family make the adjustments to kidney failure and treatment. The National Kidney Foundation affiliate and AAKP can also assist in finding help.

Should I seek counseling?

A social worker has the necessary skills and training in counseling and family therapy. If you think that counseling for you or your family members is needed, you should talk with a social worker. This professional member of the medical team can help determine if counseling can benefit you or members of your family.

How much will what I read and hear affect my adjustment?

Unfortunately, many people still believe that kidney failure is terminal, or that people with kidney failure must stay in a hospital bed, attached to a kidney machine, for 24 hours a day. A patient may start dialysis treatment, as many people do, with these beliefs. The fear and anxiety caused by expecting dialysis to be all of the horrible things you have heard and read about can cause difficulty in adjustment. The National Kidney Foundation and its affiliates work with the print and broadcast media about the realities of dialysis and kidney failure, including the fact that people who require dialysis treatment can live reasonably normal lives, have friends, work, get married, raise a family and be happy.

The best way to deal with these beliefs and myths about dialysis is for you to meet and talk with other people who are undergoing treatment for kidney failure and with the physicians, nurses, social workers and dietitians of the Renal Center.

What can the social worker do to help? A social worker can provide help in counseling services and resource and referral services. Examples of problems that may benefit from counseling services are depression and anxiety, marital and family stress, sexual concerns and concerns about death and dying. Examples of the need for resource and referral services may include inability to pay for the cost of dialysis and transplantation, hospital bills, drugs and doctor bills; lack of transportation for travel to and from dialysis treatments; and loss of employment. A social worker also functions as a patient advocate and is available to help with concerns you may have about treatment.They work as a team member with the other staff in helping you adjust to your illness.

What is rehabilitation? Rehabilitation, when the term is applied to someone who has become ill with a chronic medical condition, can mean restoring health, positive outlook, meaningful personal relationships, and rewarding activity. Vocational rehabilitation can mean restoring a patient to gainful or useful activities, including housework, childcare, and part-time or full-time jobs.

Yes. Some degree of rehabilitation is required for all people undergoing treatment for kidney failure. Restoring health, establishing a positive outlook, maintaining meaningful personal relationships and pursuing rewarding activities is part of a patient's entire adjustment process. The goal of the medical team at the dialysis unit is to rehabilitate a patient. Whether or not you require vocational rehabilitation depends on your physical health, prior occupation or ability to find a job.

Do all people with kidney failure need rehabilitation?

Most people with kidney failure can return to gainful or useful activities. It helps to have an understanding employer who accepts the fact that your life will be somewhat unstable during the initial adjustment to dialysis and that you may have to take off a few days now and then. In some cases, the type of work that you did prior to kidney failure may be too physically demanding to continue. If you have concerns about your type of work, you should talk to a physician.

Can I continue to work?

Employers, as well as the general public, need to be educated to the fact that people receiving dialysis treatment can be restored to full productivity. The myths of dialysis disability exist and need to be dealt with. Those with kidney disease qualify as handicapped under the Americans with Disabilities Act (ADA), which forbids discrimination in hiring prospective employees because of a physical handicap (see Chapter 11, *Other Questions*). As is the case with everyone, however, finding the right job can be a matter of luck,

Will I have problems finding a job?

timing and persistence. Sometimes, the biggest stumbling block to finding work is scheduled daytime dialysis treatments. A patient may request a transfer to the evening shift or to another facility that offers late afternoon or evening shifts.

Where can I find more information on vocational rehabilitation?

If you are having trouble finding a job or find that you cannot return to the type of work you were doing prior to kidney failure, you may want to seek vocational rehabilitation. For more information, you can contact a social worker or the state Department of Vocational Rehabilitation.

How can I help in my own adjustment and rehabilitation?

You can educate yourself about kidney failure and treatment. You must participate in your own care by complying with dietary regulations and medication. You should cooperate with the medical staff and report any unusual symptoms or problems that occur. You should also maintain meaningful personal relationships, communicate with your family and friends, participate in rewarding activities, set personal goals, maintain a feeling of self-worth and self-esteem and continue to live your life the best way you can in spite of kidney failure and treatment.

Financial Information and Other Resources 9

Dialysis treatment can cost between $25,000 to $30,000 per year. The average cost for kidney transplant surgery without complications is $34,000 in the United States. The federal government and some state programs provide financial assistance to help pay for the costs of treatment for kidney failure. Further information about financial assistance through the federal government is provided in this chapter.

What are the costs of treatment for chronic kidney failure?

Contact the National Kidney Foundation affiliate for information about federal assistance as well as for information on programs supported by your state.

The Medicare kidney disease provisions cover 80 percent to 100 percent of medical and hospital charges, if a patient qualifies. For example, one of the benefits of Medicare is the coverage of EPO when given in a dialysis facility. However, Medicare benefits are limited if the services are also covered by an employer group health plan. These limitations are explained later in this chapter under "What if a patient has other medical insurance?"

How can Medicare help?

You are eligible for benefits under the kidney disease provisions of Medicare if you have kidney failure *and are receiving dialysis or have a transplant* and meet one of the following qualifications:

Am I eligible for the kidney disease provisions of Medicare?

99

- You are fully or currently insured under Social Security or are entitled to a monthly Social Security or Railroad Retirement benefit
- You are the spouse or dependent child of such an individual

You are eligible for benefits under the kidney disease provisions of Medicare. If you are over 65 years of age, you may also qualify under the regular Medicare provisions for older people. Eligibility is not based on age or whether a person is currently working or unable to work.

What are the kidney disease provisions of Medicare?

The 1972 kidney disease provisions of Medicare or Public Law 92-603 were effective July 1, 1973. Since then, amendments have been made to expand the program, including the 1978 provisions of Public Law 95-292, which were effective October 1, 1978, and the Omnibus Budget Reconciliation Act of 1981, Public Law 97-35, enacted August 13, 1981. The Omnibus Budget Act of 1990 has expanded Medicare coverage of self-administered EPO for home dialysis patients effective 1991, while the Omnibus Reconciliation Act of 1993 (OBRA '93) extends immunosuppressant coverage from one year to three years.

These Medicare benefits consist of two types of insurance: Part A, or hospital insurance, and Part B, or medical insurance. Almost everyone who is eligible for Medicare is covered by hospital insurance without paying any monthly premium. Hospital insurance covers medically necessary inpatient hospital care and, under certain conditions, medically necessary post-hospital inpatient care in a skilled nursing facility, and home health care provided by a home health agency. The hospital insurance part of Medicare, for example, helps pay for an inpatient stay in an approved hospital for kidney transplant surgery. Hospital insurance has an annual deductible, and Medicare payments for services are made directly to the participating facility providing services.

When a person becomes entitled to Medicare hospital insurance because of chronic kidney failure, they are also enrolled for medical insurance or Part B of Medicare. Although they do not have to take this part of Medicare, most of the services and supplies required by chronic kidney failure are covered only by the medical insurance and not by the hospital insurance. The monthly premium for medical insurance protection covers physicians' services; outpatient hospital services; outpatient maintenance dialysis treatments in an approved dialysis facility; durable medical equipment for use in the home, such as a dialysis machine; and almost all items necessary for home dialysis, as well as many other health services and supplies. In addition to monthly premium payments, medical insurance also carries a small annual deductible payment and a 20 percent co-insurance liability.

No. The kidney disease provisions of Medicare cover a person regardless of age, if they are eligible.

Do I have to be a certain age to be eligible?

101

How can I find out if I am eligible for Medicare benefits?

The law states that you must be a Social Security or Railroad Retirement beneficiary or be "fully or currently" insured in order to be eligible for the kidney disease provisions of Medicare. You are currently insured if you have at least six quarters of coverage during the full 13-quarter period ending with the calendar quarter in which dialysis or a transplant occurs. A patient is fully insured when they have one quarter of coverage under the Social Security program for each year elapsing after 1950 (or after the year the patient attains age 21, if later) to the year in which dialysis or transplant occurs. In no case is more than 40 quarters of coverage required. The spouse or dependent child of an insured individual is also eligible. For more information on eligibility, contact the local Social Security office. A social worker can also assist in determining whether or not you are eligible for Medicare benefits.

When and how do I apply for Medicare benefits?

You should apply for Medicare benefits after the diagnosis of chronic kidney failure has been made and shortly after beginning treatment. Many people complete the application with assistance from a social worker. Also, Social Security area offices provide the necessary forms and assistance in completing them.

What is the waiting period?

Medicare coverage for dialysis treatment starts the first day of the third month after a course of dialysis is started. For example, if a person were to begin receiving dialysis treatment on May 22nd and continue treatment through the months of June and July, the

Medicare coverage would begin on August 1st. The purpose of the waiting period is to establish whether or not they have chronic kidney failure rather than acute kidney failure, which often is reversible. The Government refers to the waiting period as a qualifying period. This waiting period may be eliminated depending on the type of treatment chosen, and if this decision is made during the first three months after treatment begins. For more information on eliminating the waiting period, you should talk to a social worker. (See the section on self-care and home dialysis on page 26.)

What costs in dialysis are covered by Medicare?

Part B medical insurance helps pay for outpatient maintenance dialysis treatments in any approved dialysis facility, including the costs of laboratory tests, equipment, supplies and other services associated with treatment. Charges for maintenance dialysis vary from one approved facility to another. Medicare pays the facility based on a per treatment rate set in advance. This rate is known as the composite rate. Medicare pays 80 percent of the composite rate less any part of the Part B deductible they have not met. You are responsible for any unmet Part B deductible plus the remaining 20 percent of the composite rate. The facility may never charge more than the unmet Part B deductible plus 20 percent of its Medicare composite rate.

Physicians' services also are covered while you are receiving dialysis treatment. Medicare pays for these services through a monthly capitation payment. This amount is paid regardless of whether a patient dialyzes as an outpatient in a dialysis facility, or at home. Under this method, Medicare pays 80 percent of a physician's monthly payment less any unmet Part B deductible. A patient pays any unmet Part B deductible plus the remaining 20 percent of the monthly payment. If a physician accepts assignment, Medicare pays them directly, and you may not be charged more than the unmet Part B deductible plus 20 percent of the monthly capitation payment. (Assignment means that a physician accepts the payment approved by Medicare as the total payment.) If a physician does not accept assignment, you receive the payment and there is no limit on the amount that may be charged.

If you are admitted to a hospital because your medical condition requires the availability of other specialized hospital services on an inpatient basis, the maintenance dialysis treatments would be covered by hospital insurance, Part A, as part of the costs of the covered inpatient hospital stay. While you are in the hospital, a physician may choose to be paid for each individual service they provide. In this case, a physician receives a prorated portion of the monthly capitation payment, reduced in proportion to the number of days you are hospitalized.

What are the Medicare benefits for self-care dialysis? If people participate in a self-care training program within the first three months after treatment begins with the intention of doing self-care (home) dialysis, Medicare benefits start during the month the self-care training begins.

Yes. In addition to eliminating the waiting period if you can begin training for self-care or home dialysis within the first three months after treatment begins, Medicare covers home dialysis equipment, all necessary supplies, and a wide range of home support services. Home dialysis includes home hemodialysis, continuous ambulatory peritoneal dialysis (CAPD), continuous cycling peritoneal dialysis (CCPD) and home intermittent peritoneal dialysis (IPD). Medicare medical insurance covers rental or purchase of the dialysis equipment for home use including delivery and installation service charges. If you stop using your home dialysis equipment temporarily, for example, because you are traveling or are hospitalized, medical insurance continues payment for the equipment for up to three months after the month in which you last used it. Medicare, through the medical insurance, covers all supplies necessary to perform home dialysis, including disposable items, such as alcohol wipes, sterile drapes, rubber gloves, forceps, scissors and topical anesthetics. Drugs cannot be covered except for heparin, the heparin antidote and topical anesthetics. The medical insurance also covers periodic support services furnished by a hospital or facility, which may be necessary to assist people who remain on home dialysis. Such support services may include visits by trained hospital or facility personnel to periodically monitor their dialysis and to assist in emergencies when necessary. In addition, services of a qualified facility or hospital personnel are covered to help with the installation and maintenance of the dialysis equipment. After the

Is home dialysis covered by Medicare?

105

annual deductible is paid, Medicare pays 80 percent of all costs and services related to home dialysis treatment.

How does Medicare pay for home dialysis? There are two payment options to choose from if a person dialyzes at home: Method I or Method II. To make a choice, a person completes the Beneficiary Selection Form HCFA-382, signs it and returns it to the facility supervising their care. Once they make an initial choice, they must continue under that option until the end of the year. They can change from one Method to the other at any time by filing a new Form 382, but the change does not go into effect until the following January 1. It is important to remember that choosing Method I or Method II does not in any way prevent them from returning to treatment in a center, selecting another kind of treatment or choosing to associate with another facility. The two methods are:

Method I: The Composite Rate
Method II: Dealing Directly with Medicare

Method I: The Composite Rate

If you choose Method 1, the dialysis facility is responsible for providing all services, equipment and supplies necessary for home dialysis. Medicare pays the facility directly for these items and services at a predetermined composite rate. Under this arrangement, you are responsible for paying the annual deductible and the 20 percent coinsurance on the Medicare rate to the facility.

Method II: Dealing Directly with Medicare

If you choose Method II, you receive payment directly from Medicare for covered home dialysis equipment and supplies. Under this arrangement, you must obtain these items directly from a supplier and are responsible for paying the supplier. However, if you choose to obtain the home dialysis equipment and supplies from a facility, Medicare pays the facility directly. Whether people obtain their items from a supplier or from a facility, they are responsible for any unmet part of the annual deductible and for 20 percent co-insurance of the approved charges for these items.

Under both Methods, a person must receive home dialysis support services from a facility, for which Medicare pays the facility directly.

Is peritoneal dialysis covered by Medicare?

Yes. Peritoneal dialysis treatment in a hospital or dialysis facility has the same coverage as hemodialysis in a hospital or facility. Continuous ambulatory peritoneal dialysis (CAPD), continuous cycling peritoneal dialysis (CCPD) and home intermittent peritoneal dialysis (IPD) are covered with the same benefits as home hemodialysis.

What are the Medicare benefits for kidney transplantation?

The waiting period for Medicare benefits is waived if a person receives a kidney transplant during the waiting period. As a transplant recipient, they are eligible for Medicare Part A and Part B benefits, including coverage of costs related to:
- hospital, nursing, laboratory tests and tissue typing
- surgeon and related costs of surgery

107

- intensive care and post-surgical costs
- subsequent follow-up after transplantation
- routine costs associated with the retrieval of a donor kidney, both living related and cadaver

Medicare's hospital insurance provides 100 percent of the hospital stay and transplant operation after the annual deductible is paid. Medicare's medical insurance covers 80 percent of the cost associated with follow-up physician visits and care. Eighty percent of immunosuppressant drug expenses are covered for one year following transplantation. The Omnibus Reconciliation Act of 1993 (OBRA '93) extends immunosuppressant coverage from one year to three years for those receiving transplants after 1995. After transplantation, Medicare coverage continues for an additional 36 months and may be extended if you are disabled or unable to work. If the transplanted kidney is rejected or lost during this time, your return to dialysis is covered immediately.

Who pays for the living related donor's medical costs?

Medicare covers the full cost of medical services for a living related donor, including coinsurance and deductibles.

What if I have other medical insurance?

If there is other medical insurance, Medicare pays to the limit of its liability and the supplementary insurer generally pays that portion of the balance remaining unpaid. There is an exception, however, if the other insurance is an employer group health plan. In that case, Medicare pays only secondary benefits for a period of up to 18 months. OBRA '93 continues this until 9/30/98. During this period, the employer plan pays first for kidney dialysis and other health services. If the employer plan pays less than the amount of the provider's cost or charge, Medicare may make secondary payment to supplement the amount paid by the employer plan. At the end of the 18-month period, Medicare pays primary benefits.

Yes. You must pay the Part A hospital insurance deductible at the start of each benefit period of hospitalization as well as the Part B medical insurance annual deductible and monthly premium. You are responsible for the 20 percent co-insurance that is not covered by Part B medical insurance and all costs not covered under either plan. It may be helpful for you to talk with a social worker or dialysis unit administrator about the 20 percent coinsurance or about any other financial concerns. This can clarify any misunderstanding you have about their financial responsibilities.

Do I have to pay anything when receiving primary Medicare benefits?

If you receive a check directly from Medicare, it is intended to pay the provider of treatment, unless you have already paid for these services. In addition, the provider needs the portion attached to the Medicare check for billing purposes.

What happens if I receive a Medicare check?

The Social Security Administration office has more information on the kidney disease provisions of Medicare as does a social worker. A free publication entitled *Medicare Coverage of Kidney Dialysis and Kidney Transplant Services* is available at the Social Security Administration office.

To whom can I talk for more information about Medicare benefits?

109

What is Medicaid?

Medicaid (MediCal in California) is a federal state-supported program to pay for health care for needy and low-income residents. Medicaid benefits vary from state to state.

What is the difference between Medicare and Medicaid?

Medicare eligibility is based on a diagnosis of chronic kidney failure and on the number of quarters paid into a person's Social Security account. Eligibility for Medicaid is based on a diagnosis of chronic kidney failure and on financial need.

How can I find out if I am eligible for Medicaid?

You cannot earn more than a specified annual income to be eligible for Medicaid; this income varies from one state to another. To determine Medicaid eligibility, you should contact the county welfare department in your community. A social worker can assist in referring you to the proper Department of Public Social Service office or Social Security office for eligibility information. Pamphlets regarding Medicare are available from a social worker or the National Kidney Foundation affiliate in your area.

Are there other federal programs that can help?

Yes. A partial list with a brief description has been included below. For more information on federal programs and eligibility, you should talk with a social worker.

Veterans Administration. If you are a veteran and if the disease is service-connected, you are eligible for treatment at a VA hospital. If you do not have service-connected kidney disease, you may still be eligible for treatment at a VA hospital if the VA hospital has room in its program and chooses to provide treatment. For more information on eligibility, contact the Veterans Administration.

Social Security Disability Insurance. Social Security Disability Insurance provides a source of income for those who qualify for benefits. Qualifications include two factors: how old you are in relation to how long you have worked and the extent of your physical limitations. To qualify, you must be unable to participate in "substantial gainful activity" for a period of at least 12 months. Substantial gainful activity means that you cannot work; this must be documented by a physician's statement or by a medical facility. The first five months are not covered by disability insurance; payments begin the sixth month from the date of onset of disability. The local Social Security Administration office can provide more information.

Supplemental Security Income (SSI). If you are disabled, blind or over 65, you may be eligible to receive SSI if you meet financial eligibility criteria. Many people apply for SSI while they are awaiting their Social Security Disability. You should apply for SSI at the Social Security Administration office. It may take several months for SSI benefits to be approved.

Veterans Pensions. If you are a veteran, you may be eligible for a pension from the Veterans Administration if your income is low.

Who can help me with my finances?

A social worker can provide you with more information on financial assistance for medical expenses as well as everyday living expenses. The National Kidney Foundation affiliate can also assist you in identifying resources for financial assistance.

What organizations provide financial help?

Organizations that provide limited financial support include some affiliates of the National Kidney Foundation, the American Association of Kidney Patients (AAKP) (800) 749-2257, and the American Kidney Fund.

What is the National Kidney Foundation?

The National Kidney Foundation is the national voluntary health agency that strives to eradicate all diseases of the kidney and urinary tract and that provides services to people living with kidney disease. It supports research, public and professional education, patient and community services and public policy. The National Kidney Foundation has affiliates throughout the nation, with professional staff to service the community. Each affiliate is governed by a voluntary board of directors, and offers programs and services to meet the needs of its community. For more information on the National Kidney Foundation and the location of the closest affiliate, contact: National Kidney Foundation, 30 East 33rd St., 11th floor, New York, NY 10016, or call toll free (800) 622-9010.

What can the National Kidney Foundation do to help?

The National Kidney Foundation and its affiliates maintain information and referral services that may provide information on financial eligibility, resources and referral to other agencies that provide direct financial assistance. (Some affiliates do provide direct financial assistance.) For more information on financial assistance and services, contact the National Kidney Foundation affiliate in your local area.

What aid does the American Association of Kidney Patients (AAKP) give?

The American Association of Kidney Patients (AAKP) is the voluntary, patient organization dedicated to helping renal patients and their families deal with kidney disease through a variety of publications (*Renalife* and the *Bulletin*), educational conferences and legislative education.

What aid does the William B. Dessner Memorial Fund, Inc., give?

The William B. Dessner Memorial Fund, Inc., provides modest emergency financial aid to kidney dialysis and transplant patients at the request of their social workers. For more information, write to: The William B. Dessner Memorial Fund, Inc., 1056 Fifth Ave., #4D, New York, NY 10128.

Can the American Kidney Fund help?

The American Kidney Fund may provide direct financial assistance to people with kidney disease, including dialysis and transplant patients. Grants are based on the nature of the requirement, on urgency and on the availability of funds. For further information on eligibility and applications, contact: American Kidney Fund, 6110 Executive Blvd., Rockville, MD 20852. Call toll free (800) 638-8299.

Do I have any rights as a patient?

Yes. Included in the rules and regulations of Public Law 92-603, or the kidney disease provisions of the federal Medicare program,

113

patients or consumers do have rights as well as responsibilities. The rights and responsibilities as a patient are stated in the Federal Register, Volume 41, Number 108, adopted Thursday, June 3, 1976, and are presented, in part, as follows:

The governing body of the ESRD facility adopts written policies regarding the rights and responsibilities of patients and, through the chief executive officer, is responsible for development of, and adherence to, procedures implementing such policies. These policies and procedures are made available to patients and any guardians, next-of-kin, sponsoring agency (ies), representative payees and the public. The staff of the facility is trained and involved in the execution of such policies and procedures. The patients' rights, policies and procedures ensure at least the following:

1. Standard: informed patients. All patients in the facility:

   (a) Are fully informed of these rights and responsibilities, and of all rules and regulations governing patient conduct and responsibilities;

   (b) Are fully informed of services available in the facility and of related charges, including any charges for services not covered under title XVIII of the Social Security Act;

   (c) Are fully informed by a physician of their medical condition unless medically contraindicated (as documented in their medical records).

2. Standard: participating in planning. All patients treated in the facility:

   (a) Are afforded the opportunity to participate in the planning of their medical treatment and to refuse to participate in experimental research;

   (b) Are transferred or discharged only for medical reasons, for a patient's welfare or that of other patients, or for nonpayment of fees (except as prohibited by Title XVIII of the Social Security Act), and are given advance notice to ensure orderly transfer or discharge.

3. Standard: respect and dignity. All patients are treated with consideration, respect and full recognition of their individuality and personal needs, including the need for privacy in treatment. Provision is made for translators, where a significant number of patients experience language barriers.

4. Standard: confidentiality. All patients are ensured confidential treatment of their personal and medical records, and may approve or refuse release of such records to any individual outside the facility, except in case of their transfer to another health care institution or as required by federal, state or local law and the secretary for proper administration of the program.

5. Standard: grievance mechanism. All patients are encouraged and assisted to understand and exercise their rights. Grievances and recommended changes in policies and services may be addressed to facility staff, administration, the Network

Council and agencies or regulatory bodies with jurisdiction over the facility, through any representative of a patient's choice, without restraint or interference and without fear of discrimination or reprisal.

What is the Network Council?

Public Law 95-292 or the 1978 provisions of the Medicare program established regional "networks" for the coordination and review of dialysis and transplant facilities and programs. Each network covers an area within the United States without regard to state lines. Within each network is a coordinating council composed of individuals knowledgeable about kidney failure and treatment programs. Network offices also have paid staff members. All networks consist of a Network Coordinating Council and Medical Review Board. The function of the Network Coordinating Council, along with the Medical Review Board, is to assess the appropriateness of patient care and to assure the highest possible quality of medical care. At least one patient representative shall serve. The other members of the coordinating council include physicians and health personnel involved in the care of kidney patients. For more information on the function of the coordinating council and Medical Review Board, contact the local National Kidney Foundation affiliate.

When should I call the National Kidney Foundation?

Most affiliates of the National Kidney Foundation maintain an information and referral service during regular business hours. This service is available to any member of the community in need of information and/or referral services relating to kidney disease and treatment. Although the Foundation cannot give medical advice, it can provide written and/or verbal information on kidney disease, treatments, availability of medical services and financial assistance.

What does the National Kidney Foundation do for people with kidney disease?

National Kidney Foundation affiliates vary in the types of the programs and services they offer. In addition to maintaining an information and referral service for people with kidney disease and their families, many affiliates offer free literature on kidney diseases and methods of treatment, as well as a variety of other valuable services. For more information on the types of services offered, contact the local National Kidney Foundation affiliate.

Is the National Kidney Foundation involved in legislation and advocacy for people with kidney disease?

Yes. The National Kidney Foundation and its affiliates have supported and continue to support legislation on both a federal and state level, advocating increased benefits and support for people living with kidney and urinary tract disease and kidney failure. The National Kidney Foundation was very instrumental in passing the federal legislation, which, in 1973, enabled kidney patients to receive Medicare benefits.

Does the National Kidney Foundation support research?

Yes. The National Kidney Foundation and its affiliates have funded millions of dollars for research support to investigate the causes, prevention and treatment of kidney and urinary tract diseases and kidney failure, improvement of dialysis results, increased success rates for kidney transplantation and alternative methods of treatment for kidney failure.

What other services does the National Kidney Foundation provide?

In addition to services directed to people with kidney disease, the National Kidney Foundation and its affiliates provide professional education public education and promotion of organ donation. Some affiliates sponsor an early detection or screening program to test for asymptomatic urinary tract infections and undiagnosed high blood pressure.

What is the American Association of Kidney Patients (AAKP)?

AAKP is a voluntary organization that is dedicated to promoting the interest and welfare of people with kidney failure. It functions in all areas of kidney diseases and kidney failure and educates both the public and patients about kidney disease, care and rehabilitation. AAKP, on a national level, distributes information for patients, and promotes organ donation. AAKP also sponsors, in part, a camp program for children with kidney failure, serves as a spokesperson for kidney patients on federal legislative issues, and educates the public about kidney disease and kidney failure. Although AAKP is located in Florida, there are chapters throughout the United States, many of which are active in ongoing educational activities and social events. For more information about AAKP and the location of local chapters, call (800) 749-2257.

Are there any other organizations that provide services?

Yes. The Polycystic Kidney Research Foundation was formed for people with polycystic kidney disease and their families. This organization sponsors research and distributes information to patients and medical professionals. For more information, contact: Polycystic Kidney Research Foundation, 922 Walnut St., Kansas City, MO 64106.

118

Yes. There are many dialysis centers within the United States and internationally that accept traveling or transient people. Prior arrangements are necessary and physician approval is advised. Medicare, however, will not pay for services outside the United States.

Can I still travel if I require dialysis treatment?

Dialysis units vary in their ability to assist in travel dialysis planning. The charge nurse on the dialysis unit, the primary nurse (the one who assists in treatment or a social worker may be able to help you with the necessary paperwork and arrangements. The dialysis unit will also be asked to supply the visiting unit with individual dialysis information. If you have determined, after talking to the dialysis staff, that you have primary responsibility for making the arrangements, you should write or telephone the dialysis center at the vacation spot. Whether you write or call, you should do the following:

How do I make the necessary arrangements to travel? Who can help?

1. State name, city, and state.

2. Inform the unit where you dialyze regularly, how often and the length of each treatment.

3. Specify if you are hepatitis positive or negative and ask if the unit accepts people who are positive, negative or both. If the unit accepts positive people for example, and you are negative, you should ask to be referred to a hepatitis negative unit in the area, or to a unit that separates the positive and negative people to prevent the spread of infection. It is important that you talk to the dialysis physician about the unit's policy before making any travel arrangements.

4. Inform the unit how long you wish to dialyze there and on what dates.

What kind of information is requested by other dialysis centers?

1. *HCFA 2728:* This is the Medicare Chronic Renal Disease (CRD) Medical Evidence Report describing a person's current medical status, in codeable terms for computer storage. It is used to indicate Medicare eligibility when the visiting dialysis facility bills Medicare for treatments. Ask for a photocopy of this form from the business office of the hospital or center where you normally dialyze.

2. *Physician's Summary:* This is a medical summary of the current situation and is to be completed by the dialysis physician. It is requested to give the visiting dialysis unit an idea of a person's diagnosis, previous medical treatment and current status.

3. *Patient Information Sheet:* This sheet describes the dialysis treatments in terms of length of run, dialysis frequency, type of dialyzer used, medications, current lab values any known complications or allergies, and insurance information. Usually, the charge nurse or primary nurse assist you in completing this form.

4. *Hepatitis B Antigen Test:* This blood test verifies the hepatitis factor. Usually a person sends verification of their hepatitis status to the distant unit along with the other required dialysis information. Approximately 10 days prior to your trip, another Hepatitis B surface Antigen should be drawn; the original should be forwarded

to the distant unit and a copy should be hand-carried.

Many dialysis units, especially in areas of high tourist demand, such as Hawaii, California, Arizona, and Florida, need two or three months notice of your visit, particularly if you plan to stay longer than one or two weeks. If you plan to travel during a holiday season, you should contact the unit six months in advance. Since the units operate on first-come, first-served basis, it is advisable to make a request as early as possible. To determine where to dialyze in a travel spot, you should first check with the charge nurse or a social worker in their dialysis unit for a listing of dialysis units throughout the country. In addition, the National Kidney Foundation affiliate may have a list of dialysis units throughout the United States and other parts of the world. If you wish to have your own list of units for reference, you can write for the following:

How do I find a dialysis unit at my vacation spot?

National Listing of Providers Furnishing
Kidney Dialysis and Transplant Services
Superintendent of Documents
U.S. Government Printing Office
Washington, DC 20402

Yes. If you are currently receiving Medicare benefits, these same benefits apply toward treatment at a vacation spot within the United States. At the time you contact the dialysis unit requesting visiting dialysis, you should ask them to clarify the payment procedure. The method of payment for dialysis treatment varies from unit to unit. All dialysis units are

Will Medicare pay for my treatment when I travel?

required by law to bill Medicare for 80 percent of their allowable payment rate. Some dialysis units, particularly those located in hospitals that have large business offices, bill the supplementary insurance carrier for the remaining 20 percent. However, many units affiliated with hospitals, but not necessarily located in hospitals, ask you to pay the remaining 20 percent in cash. You should take the insurance forms from the supplemental carrier on the trip and have them filled out by the unit personnel so that there is no delay in your insurance company's reimbursement.

If you have Medicare coverage, parts A and B, and do not have a supplemental insurance policy to pick up the remaining 20 percent of your dialysis costs, you should inquire at the hospital business office to see how the 20 percent is currently being paid. If you are receiving Medicaid only and wish to travel, it is important for you to discuss this with a social worker since prior approval may be necessary before receiving guest dialysis out-of-state.

Is there anything else I should know about making travel plans?

Yes. Normally, dialysis patients from a unit in which hepatitis is present can best be accommodated by a comparable unit. While this factor may require careful planning and unit coordination and support, it is wise to be persistent in checking all available dialysis units in your desired area. Some large dialysis units in metropolitan areas may be more flexible, since they have established separate hepatitis negative and hepatitis positive dialysis units. You should talk with their dialysis physician and charge nurse regarding policy for dialysis in their unit and follow that policy.

When you arrive in the area that you are visiting, you should get settled, then call the dialysis unit to confirm the dialysis reservation and recheck the reporting time for the dialysis treatment.

Yes. There are travel agencies that assist in scheduling dialysis. Some of these agencies coordinate cruises and provide treatment during the cruise. For more information, contact the local National Kidney Foundation affiliate.

Are there any travel agencies that specialize in travel arrangements for people on dialysis?

Yes. There are several books available. Highly recommended is: *Understanding Your New Life With Dialysis*, Fourth edition, by Edith T. Oberley, M.A., and Terry D. Oberley, M.D., Ph.D. Dr. Terry Oberley is currently receiving dialysis treatment and has been for many years. This book describes his adjustment to kidney failure and dialysis, and provides a variety of useful information on kidney failure and treatment. Write to: Charles C. Thomas, 2600 South First St., Springfield, IL 62717.

Are there any books available to give me more information about kidney failure and treatment?

Ask a physician or social worker for the titles of other books on kidney failure and treatment.

Research and Kidney Failure   10

Yes. Ongoing research is being conducted throughout the United States to:

- better understand the causes of kidney diseases and kidney failure

- develop new strategies for the treatment and prevention of kidney diseases and kidney failure

- improve dialysis therapies

- increase success rates for kidney transplantation

- find alternative treatment methods for kidney failure

As a result of intensive research and technological advances, the treatment of kidney failure has changed and expanded. Many advances have made it possible for people with kidney failure to live longer and with fewer complications. Some of these research developments include:

- the use of recombinant erythropoietin to treat the anemia of chronic kidney failure. Erythropoietin has reduced the need for transfusions and has improved the exercise endurance and feeling of well-being of many people with kidney failure

- a better understanding of the immunology of transplantation that has led to the ongoing development of new medications

125

and tissue typing techniques to prevent the rejection of transplanted kidneys

- the effective use of calcitriol, the active form of Vitamin D, for the treatment of a common form of bone disease that occurs with kidney failure

- the identification of another form of bone disease in hemodialysis patients called amyloid bone disease and the development of methods to detect and diminish the accumulation of amyloid in bones and joints

- a major reduction in the occurrence of aluminum bone disease through the use of preventive interventions

- the continued improvement of continuous ambulatory peritoneal dialysis (CAPD) so that the risk of infection has been significantly reduced

Are there any recent research developments? Yes. There have been several recent research developments that have led to new ways of preventing kidney failure and treating people with kidney failure.

Recent research has demonstrated that the progression of diabetic kidney disease, a major cause of kidney failure, may be slowed by the use of blood pressure-lowering medications called angiotensin-converting enzyme (ACE) inhibitors and by very good control of the blood sugar. In addition, the use of new tests for the early detection of kidney disease in diabetic patients permits earlier intervention with preventive measures.

The development of new and more effective antihypertensive medications now offers more treatment options for people with hypertension, which remains a major cause of kidney failure.

The continued development of high-flux dialysis membranes and new biocompatible membranes has improved the efficiency and safety of hemodialysis. The development of new CAPD systems has dramatically reduced the incidence of peritonitis, the most common complication of CAPD.

Improvements in the use of immunosuppressive medications in preventing the rejection of transplantations and in tissue-type matching have increased the success rate of kidney transplantation.

Yes. Research centers throughout the United States and the world are conducting research in the treatment of people with kidney failure.

Is there promising research taking place now?

Examples of promising research include:

- development of continuous computerized monitoring of hemodialysis treatment to optimize the safety and the quality of dialysis

- improving the understanding of the interaction between the blood and hemodialyzer membranes so that even safer and more efficient membranes can be developed

- development of ways of diagnosing and treating the bone diseases associated with kidney failure

- development of portable dialyzer machines

127

- treatment of a variety of kidney diseases and conditions that can lead to chronic kidney failure

- development of new immunosuppressives, immunosuppressive strategies and tissue-typing techniques to optimize the success rate of kidney transplantation

- development of new ways of preserving donor kidneys for transplantation so that the best possible tissue matching and early function of the transplanted kidney may be achieved

Is there ongoing research that may lead to future advances in the prevention and treatment of kidney diseases and kidney failure?

Scientific studies exploring the molecular and cell biology and physiology of kidney diseases and kidney failure eventually lead to new ways of preventing and treating kidney failure. Studies on cell culture and animal models for human kidney diseases and kidney failure have produced important new insights into the many factors that contribute to the causes and complications of kidney diseases and kidney failure. Moreover, they have provided a scientific basis for developing new approaches to preventing and treating kidney failure in people.

New molecular biological techniques are being applied to the study of kidney diseases with a genetic basis and offer hope that, in the future, treatment of diseases, such as polycystic kidney disease, will become a reality. Advances in our scientific understanding of the molecular and cell biology of kidney transplantation ensure continued improvements in the success, safety and availability of kidney transplantation for people with kidney failure. Although direct clinical application of some of these scientific advances may be years in the future, new scientific explorations must be encouraged and supported so that present and future generations of people with kidney disease and kidney failure may benefit.

Where is research being done?

Research in kidney diseases and kidney failure is being conducted throughout the world. Many of the top kidney research facilities in the world are located in the United States under the supervision of internationally recognized scientists.

Who is paying for the research on kidney failure and treatment?

Most of the funding for research comes from the federal government through the National Institute of Health. The second-largest source of funding comes from the National Kidney Foundation and its affiliates throughout the United States.

How can information about the latest kidney research developments be obtained?

There are several magazines that publish information on the latest scientific research developments in kidney disease and kidney failure. One very good source is *Renalife*, which is published by AAKP. CD&N publishes the latest scientific research developments. Regional National Kidney Foundation affiliates are also a good resource for this information; anyone can request to be placed on local mailing lists for their newsletters.

Other Questions   11

Yes. Although many women on dialysis have their menstrual cycle disrupted by kidney failure, there are women who have normal pregnancies. You should wait at least one year or more after transplant before becoming pregnant, however, because renal function is more stable then. If you menstruate regularly and wish to prevent pregnancy, you should continue to protect yourself with contraceptives.

Can I still get pregnant while receiving dialysis treatment?

Yes. There are men who have fathered healthy children. Infertility may, however, be a problem if you are on dialysis.

Can I father a child while receiving dialysis treatment?

Yes. If you have no other medical complications and you are fertile, your chances of getting pregnant are the same as those for the general population of women.

Can I get pregnant after receiving a kidney transplant?

Yes. You can receive a kidney transplant from a living relative or from a deceased person. The amount of insulin required may increase as a result of the use of immunosuppressant drugs to prevent rejection, an increased appetite for food and food intake and the more efficient breakdown of insulin in your body by the new kidney. Many physi-

If I am diabetic, can I still get a transplant?

cians believe that transplantation is the preferred treatment for people who are diabetic.

What if my kidney failure is a result of polycystic kidney disease? How will I know if my children have polycystic kidney disease?

The age of onset for polycystic kidney disease varies. Statistically, half of the children of a parent with polycystic kidney disease will also have the disease. Screening of family members is a complex issue and should be discussed with your physician.

Is there a test available to determine if my unborn child has polycystic kidney disease?

No. Although the gene that causes this hereditary disease has now been identified, continued research is taking place to effectively test for this gene, during pregnancy, in the amniotic fluid.

Is exercise important?

Yes. Some degree of exercise is important for everyone to maintain health and fitness. An exercise program can help improve cardiovascular fitness, maintain flexibility and muscle strength and control weight. In addition, researchers have found a decreased incidence of depression and anxiety in those who exercise. An exercise tape, called *Easygoing Aerobics*, along with an instruction booklet, published by the National Kidney Foundation of Northern California, is available. The National Kidney Foundation affiliate can provide more information on how to order this tape. You should talk to a physician about exercise and your individual needs before beginning such a program.

Am I at risk of contracting HIV/AIDS?

Everyone is potentially at risk of transmission of HIV/AIDS (Human Immunodeficiency Virus/Acquired Immune Deficiency Syndrome). As HIV/AIDS is contracted through the exchange of body fluids, sterilization, disinfection and sanitation procedures at dialysis facilities are important. *The spread of HIV/AIDS can be prevented through careful adherence to guidelines for infection control known as universal blood and body fluid precautions that include the following for health care workers:

- wear protective gear such as gloves, scrub suits, lab coats or aprons
- wear gowns and protective eyewear and masks when blood splashes are likely
- put on a fresh pair of gloves for each direct patient encounter
- wash hands when entering the patient area, when starting or completing patient care, before leaving the work area and between patients
- dispose of needles or other sharp instruments in purchase-resistant containers located close to dialysis area
- never recap needles

Similar safety procedures are currently in use to control the spread of infection of Hepatitis B in dialysis units. The HIV/AIDS virus is spread much less readily than Hepatitis B in dialysis units because the blood of a person infected with HIV/AIDS has fewer infectious viral particles than does the blood of someone with Hepatitis B. In addition, all blood donations are being screened for the

133

HIV/AIDS antibody making any blood transfusion as safe as possible.

*U.S. Department of Health and Human Services booklet
AIDS Information For The Dialysis Professional*

What is aluminum intoxication?

Aluminum intoxication is the buildup of aluminum in the body, which can cause dialysis dementia and aluminum bone disease. Some of the early signs of dialysis dementia include slurring of words and difficulty in speaking, jerking muscle movements and loss of memory or impaired thinking. These symptoms may result from other causes unrelated to aluminum intoxication. However, if you experience any of these symptoms, it is important to discuss them with a physician. Aluminum bone disease is caused by the buildup of aluminum in the body, which may prevent normal bone formation. Treatment for aluminum intoxication includes chelation therapy, which involves receiving an intravenous medication before or during dialysis; and reduction of exposure to aluminum from water, phosphate binders and food preparation, since prevention is possible and wise.

Are there standards for dialyzer reuse?

Standards and guidelines for the safe reuse or reprocessing of hemodialyzers have been developed by organizations, including the National Kidney Foundation, AAKP and other medical and scientific organizations. The Federal government requires that all treatment facilities receiving Medicare reimbursement comply with standards and conditions of participation for safe and effective dialyzer reuse and processing.

Some tap water contains disinfectant called chloramines, which are a combination of chlorine and a small amount of ammonia. Chloramines are toxic and must be removed from water used in the artificial kidney machine. The dialysis unit takes special precautions to remove chloramines from the water. If a person dialyzes at home, the water must be treated using one of a variety of methods available. Not all tap water contains chloramine, however, so they should check with the dialysis unit to see if this is the case in their area.

What are chloramines?

Yes. The National Kidney Foundation of Arizona offers a book in Spanish called, *Buscando Respuestas*. A Spanish version of *When Your Kidneys Fail*, called *Cuando Sus Riñones Fallan*, is also available. For more information on either of these books, contact the National Kidney Foundation affiliate.

Is there information on kidney failure in Spanish?

The Americans with Disabilities Act (ADA) is a federal law effective July 26, 1992, which forbids discrimination against people with disabilities. Anyone with renal failure, whether treated by hemodialysis, peritoneal dialysis or successfully transplanted, qualifies as disabled and is covered under this law. There are exclusions if you are a drug or alcohol abuser unless you have completed or are in a drug rehabilitation program and have ceased drinking or using illegal drugs. The act covers employment, transportation, and public accommodation. This section discusses the employment-related aspects of the ADA.

Is there any protection against employment discrimination for renal patients?

Which employers are affected by the ADA?

All public and private employers who employ 25 or more people for more than 20 weeks *in the current or preceding year* are included as of July 26, 1992. As of July 26, 1994, all employers employing 15 or more people for more than 20 weeks *in the current or preceding year* are covered. The United States government, Indian tribes and private membership clubs are not covered; however, the United States government provides similar rights under the Rehabilitation Act of 1973 (29 U.S.C. 706).

What must employers do to comply?

Under the law, employers can only consider the individual's ability to do the job. They are not required to lower standards of production quality or quantity and may choose the most highly qualified applicant. In doing this, employers must make "reasonable accommodation," which includes:

"(A) making existing facilities used by employees readily accessible and usable by individuals with disabilities; and

(B) job restructuring, part-time or modified work schedule, reassignment to a vacant position, acquisition or modification of existing equipment or devices, appropriate adjustment or modifications of examination, training materials, or policies, the provision of qualified readers or interpreters and other similar accommodations for individuals with disabilities." [1] [2]

Employers can be excused from accommodation if it causes undue hardship, taking into

[1] Americans with Disabilities Act of 1990. Pub. L.101-335, sec. 3/2.
[2] Ibid. sec 101.9.

consideration the:

- nature of the accommodation
- cost to provide the accommodation
- company's financial resources
- size of the company

An accommodation for a renal patient may be to allow for flexible hours to accommodate the dialysis schedule or CAPD exchanges. The time used, however, may have to be made up. *Under some circumstances, flexible hours might be an undue hardship for an employer and thus unavailable as an accommodation.*

Employers are prohibited by the ADA from requiring a pre-employment medical examination. They can require an examination after the job has been offered, if it is required of all new employees in the same or similar positions. Drug testing is also allowed if required of all new employees.

What if I am asked to have a pre-employment physical examination?

Except for in a post-job offer medical exam, you may be asked only those questions that are job-related and regarding your ability to perform the job. You may not be questioned regarding your disability or its severity. If asked any questions specifically regarding health or disability, you may choose to discuss it only with regard to your ability to do the job.

What if I am asked about my health status?

Employers may not retaliate if you make a charge against an employer, testify or in any way exercise your right granted under this Act.

What are an employer's rights?

137

To whom can I talk if I feel discriminated against by an employer or prospective employer? You can contact the Equal Employment Opportunity Commission (listed under United States Government in the telephone book). State and local legal resources are also listed in the telephone book and may be able to assist. A unit social worker is another resource for information, assistance, referral and advocacy.

Advance Directives   **12**

Making Medical Decisions, Limiting Undesired Treatment, and Using a Living Will or Durable Power of Attorney to Ensure Your Treatment Preferences Are Respected

In medicine or health care, patients and health care professionals need to ask several questions: What is wrong? What can be done? What should be done? Who should decide?

In answering these questions, it is helpful to be mindful of the *goals of medicine*:

- to maintain or restore health and prevent or cure illness
- to prevent suffering and relieve pain
- to reduce impairment and restore function
- to preserve the quality as well as the extent of life

Health care professionals need to know the patient as person, to know their beliefs, values, attitudes and preferences.

This chapter explains *advance directives* (statements made by an individual to guide their treatment or to indicate whom they would like to make decisions for them should they ever become unable to). To understand advance directives, it is essential first to understand how decisions are made for competent and for incompetent individuals. In general, doctors recommend and patients decide (but if someone has lost the ability to decide, their loved ones can make decisions for them). In order to understand advance directives, you should also know that patients have the right to limit or to refuse as well as to consent to treatment. When illness is excessively burdensome or is futile, it is often a patient or their family who initiate considerations to limit treatment.

Medical Decision-making: A Responsibility Shared Between Doctor and Patient

What is decision-making capacity (competence)?

Decision-making capacity (or competence) is the ability to make decisions for yourself, and this requires the ability to understand your illness, the expected consequences of the illness, and the nature, probable outcome, and possible risks of the proposed treatment and of alternative treatments. An individual needs the ability to reason about the alternatives, to weigh their benefits and burdens and to choose among them.

What is informed decision-making (informed consent or refusal)?

Informed consent (or refusal) is the legal right to make health care decisions for yourself (and to be provided the information necessary to do so). This right stems from the ethical principle of autonomy (the right of competent individuals to determine what will be done to their own bodies).

What is required for informed consent?

The information required for informed consent is the nature and prognosis of the illness, the benefits and risks of possible treatments and the consequences of forgoing treatment. In addition, competent, informed health care deci-sion-making requires freedom from duress or coercion, recognition of your values and goals, receipt of adequate, understandable medical information and the ability to understand it and to reason about the options and consequences. Furthermore, health care professionals are appreciative when patients are able and willing to communicate their preferences and deci-sions and to explain them.

Patients are constrained in informed consent when they are provided inadequate informa-tion, unexplained information, excessive information *(information overload)*, irrele-vant information or distorted information. Other factors that impair or preclude informed consent are the use of technical jargon by health care professionals, irrationality or immaturity of the patient, fear or other controlling influences, and coercion or manip-ulation by the health care professional, family, or friends (even though their intent is to help the patient).

Are there constraints upon patient comprehension in informed consent?

Limiting Treatment: You May Find the Burdens of Illness and Treatment Exceed the Benefits

Yes. In the case of Nancy Beth Cruzan (a young Missouri woman who was permanently unconscious following an automobile accident), the U.S. Supreme Court stated that there is a constitutional right to refuse treatment, includ-ing artificial nutrition and hydration; that this right is not lost if a person becomes incompe-tent (it may then be exercised by a surrogate);

May I refuse treatment, even life-sustaining treatment?

141

and this right does not require that one have a terminal condition. The aspect of the ruling in Cruzan that led many people to execute advance directives was the holding that a state may require clear and convincing evidence of a patient's wishes.

Why might I forgo life-sustaining treatment?

Treatment might be omitted because it is ineffective, dangerous, expensive or simply because it is not your desire.

Is there a difference between withdrawing and withholding treatment?

Although ethically and legally there is no difference between withdrawing treatment and withholding it (never starting it), it is usually much more difficult emotionally to withdraw than to withhold treatment. On the other hand, it is very important for health care professionals and for relatives and loved ones to be willing to allow you to discontinue treatment if, after a trial or a prolonged course of treatment, you feel the treatment is not beneficial or find the burden of the illness and of continued treatment outweighs the benefits.

What is CPR?

"CPR" stands for CardioPulmonary Resuscitation. It is the coordinated set of treatments that can be given when the heart and/or lungs suddenly cease to function; that is, when a person has a cardiac (heart) or pulmonary (lung) arrest. CPR consists of breathing for the patient via a mask or via a tube in the windpipe and compressing the chest to "massage" the heart to pump blood throughout their body. Medications may also be given.

When a person has a cardiac arrest and/or pulmonary arrest, they promptly lose consciousness and are unable either to consent to or refuse CPR. Some people who are terminally ill, however, or who suffer physically and/or mentally wish not to be resuscitated should they have an arrest, and they can request in advance not to have CPR should an arrest occur.

Can I refuse CPR? And why might I wish to do so?

A *DNR*, or *Do Not Resuscitate*, order is an order written in a patient's chart to alert health care professionals to honor their preference not to have CPR.

What is a DNR order?

Certainly, you may request treatment even though it was not recommended or offered spontaneously by a physician or other health care personnel. If the request is reasonable, surely treatment will be provided. A potential conflict may occur, however, if you or your family believe the request appropriate, but physicians or other health care professionals do not. A physician's professional medical ethic (to do good, to do no harm and to allow people to choose from among effective, beneficial treatments) does not entitle a patient to harmful, ineffective, or inappropriate treatment. The problem may be, however, that you judge the requested treatment to be appropriate, but a physician believes it is not.

Since I can refuse treatment, can I demand it?

In the overwhelming majority of health care decisions, physicians and patients agree. At times, there are different opinions about what you need, about different goals for treatment, or even about different moral beliefs. Such

What if the doctor and I (or family) disagree?

143

disputes may resolve with discussion or nego-
tiation and compromise or with new insights
provided by consultation with other health
care professionals or with an ethics commit-
tee. At times, you must transfer to another
physician.

Decision-Making for Those Who Lack Decision-making Capacity

What is incompetence? Incompetence in its broad sense is a lack of decision-making capacity. Some restrict the word to its narrow or legal sense: a lack of decision-making ability determined by a court. Yet, another legal meaning of the word is not having reached the age of majority at which one is legally entitled to make health care decisions for oneself.

What are the criteria for incompetence? Health care professionals and family and friends (as well as judges) may reasonably conclude a person is incompetent if they cannot understand their disclosed situation, analyze risks and benefits, state a preference or make a "reasonable" choice or decision. The latter is, of course, a dangerous basis for concluding someone incompetent, since individuals have the right to idiosyncratic beliefs, preferences and choices.

How can decisions be made for incompetent patients? In the past, physicians paternalistically made unilateral decisions regarding the care of incompetent patients. They prescribed what, in their judgment, was in the best interest of this person. Advancing medical technology now allows many treatments that not all people would want. Furthermore, our belief that people have the right to be informed and to make decisions for themselves requires that someone other than a health care professional speak on behalf of an incompetent person. A proxy or surrogate should consent to, or refuse, recommendations made by a physician.

A proxy (literally a person who cares for another's interests) or surrogate (literally one who is asked for, or who is a substitute) is a person authorized or appointed to act for another. The two words may be used interchangeably. In some states, the hierarchy of individuals who may legally serve as surrogates is defined by statutory law, in others by common law (that is, by the precedent of court-decided cases).

What is a proxy or a surrogate decision-maker?

Commonly, the proxy or surrogate with legal priority or highest standing is either an attorney-in-fact (see page 147) appointed in a durable power of attorney or a conservator or guardian appointed by a court. Next is a spouse, followed by a parent or adult child, and then a sibling; only thereafter come more distant relatives, caretakers and friends. In many jurisdictions, however, under emergency circumstances, a physician, or two physicians, may make decisions without approval by a surrogate.

Who is the legal proxy?

A morally valid surrogate or proxy is someone who has significant involvement with an individual, knowledge of their values, willingness

Who is a morally valid proxy?

145

to express their values or wishes, and no emotional conflicts or other conflicts of interest that would interfere with making appropriate decisions for that person.

How do proxies (surrogates) make decisions for incompetent patients? For incompetent patients, the doctor recommends and the patient's proxy decides. In the case of a decision by a proxy or surrogate, however, it is very important that the surrogate state not what they would want, but rather *what the patient would want*. Under ideal circumstances, a patient would have informed the surrogate what they would want under the specific circumstances that pertain now. These are called the *express* or *expressed wishes* of a patient.

Unfortunately, most of us cannot predict accurately what circumstances will befall us, and, thus, few of us have informed our proxy (or agent-in-fact under a durable power of attorney for health care) specifically what we would want. Under such circumstances, a proxy must make an educated guess that we call a *substituted judgment*. This determination may be based on a statement a patient made in the past about someone else in similar circumstances or it may be based upon knowledge of a patient's values, beliefs or attitudes in general. When neither an express wish is known nor a reasonable substituted judgment can be made, the proxy must make a judgment based on the *best interests* of the patient. This best interest judgment should be from the perspective of the patient.

Unfortunately, substituted and best interests judgments are not perfect. Relatives sometimes overestimate, and at other times underestimate, what treatment this person would want. In the absence of clear treatment directives or express wishes, proxy judgments are the best we have for incompetent patients (and are somewhat closer to what patients would want than are judgments by physicians).

What is an agent, agent-in-fact or attorney-in-fact?

These terms are interchangeable. An *agent-in-fact* or an *attorney-in-fact* is a person officially appointed or designated in writing by an individual to act on their behalf. The word *attorney* does not mean a lawyer or attorney-at-law, but simply a person given authority to act by and for another person. The document authorizing this agency is called a *power of attorney*. It is durable, since it becomes or remains effective in the event the individual becomes disabled or incompetent.

The durable power of attorney for health care is specific in granting the agent or attorney-in-fact the authority to make health care decisions (but not financial or other decisions). It becomes effective only when a person is no longer competent.

Advance Directives: Planning in Advance to Ensure Your Values are Respected and Preferences Honored Even If You Lose the Ability to Make Health Care Decisions

What is an advance directive?

An *advance directive* (not an advanced directive), is a statement made in advance of becoming incompetent that either specifies what treatment a person would or would not

147

want under certain circumstances (a *treatment directive*) or specifies who should make those decisions (a *proxy directive*), or both.

A *treatment directive* is a statement made to direct one's treatment after one becomes incompetent. Most often treatment directives are written to limit rather than to request care, but either is acceptable.

A *proxy directive* states whom one wants to make decisions for them in the event of their loss of decision-making capacity.

A *comprehensive directive* is a combined directive that both indicates treatment preferences and appoints a proxy (or successor proxies if the initial proxy should be unable or unwilling to serve).

Is a DNR request an advance directive?
Yes and no. Conceptually, a request for a DNR order *is* an advance treatment directive. In practice, however, a request for a DNR order is not usually thought of as an advance directive. Probably the reason is that all other treatment and proxy directives are durable; that is, they last permanently (or for a number of years, as specified in the statutes of various states). In contrast, a DNR order lasts only for the specific hospitalization or stay in a long-term-care facility, and must be rewritten for each admission if a patient and physician want it to continue.

Should DNR orders and advance directives be reviewed?
For all people whose health or life circumstances change materially, a DNR should be reconsidered and either reaffirmed or suspended. This is true for all advance directives; they should be reviewed periodically

and whenever the health or life circumstances of a person changes.

A living will is a treatment directive, usually a treatment-limitation directive. In the narrow sense, a living will is a brief, often generic or standardized statement, such as the following:

What is a living will?

"If the situation should arise in which there is no reasonable expectation that I will recover from an incapacitating physical disability or mental infirmity, I request that I be allowed to die and not be kept alive by artificial means or heroic measures."

In the broad sense, a living will is any statement (commonly written rather than oral) by a competent individual regarding his preference for treatment or treatment limitation or regarding who should make such decisions should the individual become incapacitated. It is called a *living* will, because unlike a normal testamentary or property will, which becomes effective only after death, a living will becomes effective during one's life, though only after one has become unable to speak competently for him- or herself.

The above example of a living will is a poor example of a treatment directive, however. Although such a simple, general statement may seem clear to an individual (who in their own mind personalizes its words to their own circumstances), it is much too vague to direct others (such as one's physician or health care providers or even one's loved ones) unless it is accompanied by detailed discussion (or knowledge) of one's values, beliefs, attitudes and preferences. What is a *reasonable*

149

expectation, or *recovery*, or *incapacitating physical disability*, or what are *artificial means* or *heroic measures* to one person is/are not to another. A good living will is more specific, even if goals, values and preferences are stated in general terms.

What is a Durable Power of Attorney for Health Care (DPAHC)?

A durable power of attorney for health care is a written document that appoints another individual (or successor individuals) as proxy to make health care decisions on behalf of the person or principal. It becomes effective only upon the principal's loss of ability to make decisions for themselves. It is durable in the sense that it remains valid indefinitely or at least for a number of years. Many believe this is the best type of advance directive because it allows you to appoint any adult in whom you have great confidence to make appropriate decisions in the future under circumstances that can rarely be foreseen with sufficient certainty or detail allows you to make those decisions clearly and specifically for your future.

What is the Natural Death Act?

The Natural Death Act is legislation that allows you to direct a physician to withhold or withdraw life-sustaining treatment (and thereby to allow a *natural* death) in the event of terminal illness, sometimes with the additional requirement of disability or infirmity. Such legislation was the first statutory advance directive (California, 1976), and it provided immunity to a physician and hospital who withheld or withdrew life-sustaining treatment. Unfortunately, this statute was uncommonly used in its initial formulation because it required that before one could even execute the document, one had to have been notified 14 or more days previously of a terminal condition attested to in writing by two physicians. In California, the law has been amended to allow any competent adult to execute the declaration in advance of illness (though it becomes effective only upon diagnosis of a terminal condition or permanent unconsciousness). It still applies, however, only if there is a terminal condition or permanent unconsciousness, restrictions not present in many states' living will and durable power statutes. Nevertheless, this document can be used instead of a durable power of attorney for those who do not trust another individual to make health care decisions or prefer not to burden anyone to do so.

Are advance directives legal documents?

Most states have enacted legislation legalizing treatment directives (living wills) and/or proxy directives (durable powers of attorney). Even in states that do not have such legislation, case law or other precedents recognize the rights of individuals to direct their own care and to have surrogate decision-makers, rights determined to be constitutional by the U.S. Supreme Court. Written information concerning state laws (both statutory and court-determined) regarding these rights and advance directives (as well as hospital policies regarding such rights) are available at virtually all hospitals in the United States.

Since the overwhelming majority of physicians and hospitals want to respect the rights of patients to name a proxy or to forgo treatment when it is viewed as more burdensome than beneficial, the legality of advance directives is more a technicality than a necessity. The important thing is that patients discuss these matters with their physicians *and* with their loved ones (*especially* with the person they wish to be their proxy).

Do I need an attorney to draw up an advance directive?

No. Although it is permissible, it is not necessary. There are many forms available throughout the United States. Not all of them are legally acceptable, however, so if legality is desired, you should be sure to obtain the appropriate form for your state of residence. A social worker in your dialysis unit or renal center should be able to advise you where to obtain forms, and may be very helpful in discussing your particular circumstances and the advisability of executing an advance directive. Witnessing by a notary or other appropriate witness (es) is necessary for the directive to be legal.

What is the Patient Self-Determination Act (PSDA)?

The PSDA is a federal statute requiring hospitals, long-term care facilities, hospice programs, home health agencies and prepaid health plans (HMOs) to provide written information:

- upon admission concerning one's rights under state law to accept or to refuse treatment and to formulate advance directives
- concerning the policies of the provider or organization respecting the implementation of such rights

and to:

- comply with state law respecting advance directives
- not condition care on execution of an advance directive
- document whether or not a patient has an advance directive
- educate hospital staff and community on issues concerning advance directives

The time of admission to a hospital, nursing home, hospice or dialysis facility is not ideal for considering all of the circumstances and issues basic to formulating an advance directive since it is invariably an emotionally challenging (even if not a physically disabling) time. Thus, it is preferable that you and your physician discuss advance directives in advance of hospitalization or dialysis (and in advance of their need).

If you have a valid advance directive, a copy should be obtained at the time of admission to a dialysis facility. If not, since the initiation of dialysis is overwhelming for many people, the National Kidney Foundation recommends that unless you indicate a desire for further discussion at the time of admission you should be provided information within a month of initiation of dialysis. If a patient does not wish to discuss or execute an advance directive at that time, the National Kidney Foundation suggests the patient be approached again, within three months, when "the patient has reached a level of comfort with dialysis and with the staff."

153

What is the benefit of having an advance directive?

Probably the greatest benefit of having an advance directive is having thought about your health and illness and treatment options in relation to your values, goals and your preferences. This should also trigger discussing these matters with your physician and with your family and friends. Even if a legal document is not completed or preferences written out, such discussions go a long way to protect your right to have or to refuse treatment by your own choice should you lose the ability to speak for yourself. Furthermore, it greatly reduces the burden on your family and your physician who would have to make decisions for you if you become too ill to do so for yourself and to know your treatment preferences and whom you wish to make decisions for you. It also provides the physician and the proxy with legal protection when they follow your wishes.

Are there disadvantages of having an advance directive?

Unfortunately, there are potential disadvantages of having an advance directive. Sometimes, professionals, relatives, or friends who only know you have one, but do not know what it contains, jump to the conclusion that you do not want life-sustaining treatment, even if your directive indicates you would, or even if the directive simply names whom you want to make decisions for you. Another potential disadvantage is that you may fail to update the advance directive when you change your mind concerning either treatment or proxy preferences.

Yet another disadvantage occurs if your treatment directive is poorly or vaguely written and inadequately clarified in discussions with your physician and/or health care proxy. Discussion is probably the most important component of a health care directive. It often helps to clarify your own understanding of your illness, treatment options and prognosis, as well as to clarify and articulate your beliefs, values and preferences, particularly those that influence decisions about your health care. In turn, this helps you communicate your wishes clearly to your physician, proxy and loved ones.

The University of New Mexico's Center for Health Law and Ethics developed a series of questions (which the developers call a "values history") for public guardians to use to ask friends of solitary, incapacitated patients what this person believed or had said about their beliefs, values, health and treatment preferences in order to guide the guardian to make appropriate decisions for an incompetent individual patient who had no other surrogate. As the values history was being developed, it became clear it could be helpful to anyone, not just the designated guardian, to obtain insight into or to clarify their own values, to articulate them, and preferably to record them for use by a surrogate should they become decisionally incapacitated.

What is a values history?

Questions in the values history ask about your living environment; your family and friends; your religious background and beliefs; your attitudes toward life in general and toward independence and control, health, doctors, illness, death and dying, and finances. They ask whether you have wishes regarding specific medical procedures, such as dialysis, artificial ventilation, artificial nutrition and hydration and organ donation, and regarding a funeral, eulogy and obituary. The questions also ask if you have any written documents, particularly advance directives.

Can I be required to have an advance directive?

No. The Patient Self-Determination Act, a federal law, specifically prohibits health care facilities or providers from conditioning admission or provision of insurance or services upon whether or not you have executed an advance directive.

Why do so few people have advance directives?

Many individuals do not know what an advance directive is, or if they know, do not realize it would be appropriate for them to have. Many others do not have an advance directive because the subject raises unpleasant or frightening issues.

Doubtless, more individuals will wish to have an advance directive when they understand how valuable it can be in protecting their right to make health decisions for themselves, and when they consider how helpful it is to their loved ones and physician to know their preferences for health care. This is particularly important for patients with chronic illness.

Why should a dialysis patient have an advance directive?

For the same reasons that everyone should have one—and for additional reasons. Dialysis is very effective in prolonging lives of those who would otherwise die of kidney failure. Fortunately, the quality of health and life for the great majority of people on dialysis is acceptable and for many substantially better than that. Most people are able to work and can do most of the activities they wish to do, but as many as 10 percent of chronic dialysis patients discontinue dialysis because the burdens of illness and treatment outweigh the benefits of continuing to live. Perhaps half of those who discontinue dialysis are no longer able to make decisions for themselves at the time dialysis is discontinued because of intercurrent illness with altered consciousness or because of dementia.

By having an advance directive, they are assured of having their own preferences for health care respected, including the continuation of dialysis or of other life-sustaining treatment if that is their preference (or discontinuation, if that is their choice). Furthermore, it is a great relief to family members and to physicians to know a patient's preferences and to feel secure that they are doing what this person would have wanted.

Why do some people forgo or stop dialysis?

Specific reasons some people elect not to start dialysis (when they are approaching end-stage renal failure) or elect to stop dialysis (even when they have done well on it in the past) are:

- the presence or development of unrelated disease that causes unrelenting pain and suffering (such as widespread cancer), extreme physical disability (such as a severe stroke or multiple amputations), or will cause a difficult death in a very short period of time
- such severe dementia that they are unable to relate to others or to understand their own illness and the necessary dialysis treatment (e.g., dementia from Alzheimer's

157

disease or from multiple strokes)
- the occurrence of such severe brain injury that they are permanently unconscious (e.g., from an automobile accident or from a cardiac or pulmonary arrest)

Fortunately, these various conditions, with rare exception (such as a stroke in a dialysis patient with uncontrolled hypertension or blindness and amputations in a severe diabetic), are no more common in patients with end-stage renal disease. They do occur, however, just as they do in other people or in otherwise healthy individuals, and one should prepare for unexpected as well as for foreseeable problems.

Why should a person with a transplant have an advance directive?

For the same reasons that everyone should have one—and for additional reasons. People other than those whose kidney donor is an identical twin are susceptible to rejection of the transplanted kidney and need to take powerful anti-rejection medications that may cause a number of complications. If the transplanted kidney is attacked by your body's defenses against foreign substances, and if this rejection cannot be reversed, you must return to dialysis (and thus should have an advance directive, just as all patients should). Anti-rejection medications increase the risk of infection. Serious infections may impair decision-making capacity; e.g., confusion from meningitis or delirium from any infection with very high fever or very low blood pressure. And if, at that time, major decisions need to be made, it would be helpful if you had an advance directive, at least one designating your preferred proxy, who hopefully would know what decisions you would prefer.

Transplant patients may have uncontrolled high blood pressure, and, thus, like dialysis patients, they are somewhat more susceptible to strokes that could impair their understanding or their ability to communicate preferences, and that could potentially cause paralysis or other serious physical impairment.

Can a teenager have an advance directive?

Although advance directives are not generally legal if made before age 18, they are certainly helpful to health care professionals caring for teenagers or children and to parents who must make major health care decisions for their child. So long as a patient can understand, reason, and express their preferences, and so long as they are not depressed or under duress or coercion, statements about preferences for treatment or for surrogates are ethically valid and should be respected.

What should be included in a good advance directive?

There is diversity of opinion regarding this question, and a good advance directive for one individual may be different from a good directive for another. Some believe one should have only a proxy directive and not a treatment directive because it is so difficult to imagine which of the many potential complications of a known specific illness one may develop.

Others believe treatment directives are helpful so long as they are general enough to guide a physician and proxy, but not so specific as to constrain or restrict their making decisions for you that you might make differently than stated in the advance directive because of unexpected complications of the illness or its treatment, different coexistent conditions or

159

changes in the context that you could not have predicted.

Still, others believe treatment directives should be as specific as possible stating not only your goals for treatment, but also your values, where you would wish to be treated, and specific preferences for treatment in a variety of specific, but albeit hypothetical, circumstances. They also suggest you indicate how much leeway, if any, you would wish to give your proxy and physician to override your stated treatment preference if the proxy and the physician thought your previously stated preference was not in your best interest or was no longer what you would choose (e.g., because your circumstances had changed or because a new treatment had become available for the condition requiring treatment).

Where can I get help in learning about advance directives or in preparing one?

Since the Patient Self-Determination Act became law, health care professionals of all disciplines have become increasingly knowledgeable about advance directives. Furthermore, written materials and even audio-visual tapes (including some prepared for dialysis professionals and patients) have become available. Virtually all hospitals, nursing homes, hospice programs, home health agencies and prepaid health plans have written materials available for those they attend. So, too, does Choice in Dying, the National Council for the Right to Die (200 Varick Street, New York, NY 10014-4810, (800) 989-9455). Some Health Decisions organizations hold workshops to educate the public and to assist you to fill out advance directives (e.g., California Health Decisions, 505 S. Main Street, Suite 400, Orange, CA 92668, (714) 647-4920). The National Kidney Foundation has prepared materials on advance directives to assist dialysis units and dialysis health care professionals as well as a brochure to educate patients, and these are available from affiliate organizations throughout the United States.

Regarding the components of a good advance directive noted in the preceding section, most are discussed in greater detail in the writings of Linda and Ezekiel Emanual (e.g., an article in the Journal of the American Geriatrics Society, Volume 39, page 1221 in 1991). Regarding the suggestion for flexibility or leeway in advance directives, a study of dialysis patients was reported in the Journal of the American Medical Association, Volume 267, page 59, 1992. Some of the suggestions of these authors (for the most part from these articles) are outlined below:

Linda Emanual suggests that goals of treatment may be specified by checking one of the following statements:

- Prolong life and treat everything
- Attempt cure, but reevaluate often
- Value the quality of life more than the duration of life
- Provide comfort care only

You may also write your own goals in your own words for the advance directive.

The Emanuals have developed scenarios or vignettes that are examples of very serious conditions that patients might develop. They suggest that patients check off each of the above-stated goals with what they would wish for in each of the following scenarios:

- coma or permanent unconsciousness with no hope of recovery
- coma with a small chance of recovery, greater chance of brain damage and a still greater chance of not recovering
- inability to recognize people, speak meaningfully or live independently, and a terminal illness
- the same but without a terminal illness
- chronic illness with mental disability or physical suffering and development of an acute life-threatening, but reversible illness
- one's current state of health and development of an acute life-threatening, but reversible illness

A person can also indicate where they wish to be treated for a new, acute, serious ailment (or for each of the preceding six scenarios): in an acute care hospital, in a nursing home, in a hospice institution, or at home (with or without the attendance of home health nurses, social workers or hospice professionals).

It is wise for people to specify the leeway to override stated treatment preferences that they would wish to grant a proxy and physician if they both agreed that the stated preference was no longer in this person's best interest (e.g., because of a change in their circumstances, or because a new treatment has become available). A person might indicate no leeway, a little, a lot or complete leeway.

If you decide to make an advance directive, whether it be a formal, legal, written document or an informal, oral statement, you must be sure to communicate your preferences to your chosen proxy, to others who are seriously concerned with your welfare and who would respect your preferences, and to the physician(s). If you have written documents, you should provide your proxy, your family, your physician, the hospital, and the dialysis unit with copies, and take a copy with you when traveling.

Can advance directives be changed or rescinded?

Yes. You should reconsider your treatment preferences and update your advance directive (write a new one, or change, suspend, or cancel the old one) whenever circumstances change (or whenever you wish to do so). If you change your advance directive, you must remember to inform your changes to your proxy, family, physician, hospital and dialysis unit, preferably in writing. Also, you must be sure to draw a line through your old advance directive, write on it that it has been changed or revoked, and date and sign your statement.

You can't change an advance directive if you do not have one, however. If that is the case, now is the time to ensure your future. If you do have an advance directive, it may already be time for you to update it.

This chapter was written by Ronald B. Miller, M.D., a nephrologist who is Clinical Professor of Medicine and Director of the Program in Medical Ethics at the University of California, Irvine, and who is Clinical Consultant and Chairman of the Scientific Advisory Board of Spectra Laboratories, Inc., a national ESRD laboratory in Fremont, California. He was a former chairman of the Scientific Advisory Council of the National Kidney Foundation of Southern California.

GLOSSARY

Acquired immune deficiency syndrome (AIDS): The multiplicity of implications that may follow a viral infection that attacks the body's immune system, making the patient unable to fight off other serious infections.

Acute kidney failure: A sudden and severe, usually temporary, failure of kidney function that can occur during a period of a few hours or days, and may last days, weeks or even months.

Advance directive: A statement made by an individual to guide his or her treatment or to indicate whom the individual would like to make health care decisions for him or her should he or she become unable to make decisions.

Agent, Agent-in-fact, Attorney-in-fact: These three terms are interchangeable. They name the person officially appointed or designated in writing by an individual to act on his or her behalf should he or she become incapable of making health care decisions.

Allergic: Being unusually sensitive to a particular substance (for example, a drug, grass or food).

Aluminum intoxication: The buildup of aluminum in the body, which can cause a disorder called dialysis dementia or aluminum bone disease.

Analgesics: Medications that relieve pain and, in some cases, reduce fever.

Anemia: A condition that is caused by the lack of sufficient red blood cells in the body and can cause one to be tired or weak as a result.

Anemic: Having anemia or less than the normal number of red cells in the blood.

Angina: Chest pain caused by a reduced blood supply to the heart muscle.

Antacid: Medications that block or neutralize stomach acid, some of which are also used as phosphate binders.

165

Antibiotics: Medications that either stop the growth of bacteria or kill bacteria.

Antibody: A body substance that fights off disease and foreign substances or reacts against body tissues.

Anticoagulants: A type of medication that prevents blood from clotting.

Artery: Vessel carrying blood away from the heart.

Artificial kidney: Refers to dialyzer.

Artificial kidney machine: Refers to a hemodialysis machine through which a patient's blood is circulated in order to maintain the chemical and fluid balance of the body.

Artificial kidney treatment: Process of maintaining the chemical balance of the blood when the kidneys have failed. Usually refers to hemodialysis.

Bacteria: Refers to germs.

Best interests: A judgment as to what treatment would be best for a patient who has become incompetent, or the judgment made by a proxy or surrogate to the best of the proxy's ability from the perspective of the patient, which is what the proxy judges the patient would believe was in the patient's own best interest.

Biotechnology: Using biology to solve problems relating to humans and disease; see also recombinant DNA technology.

Bladder: The sac in which urine produced by the kidneys is collected and stored until the urine is released from the body.

Blood flow rate: The rate at which blood flows through the dialyzer.

Blood leaks: Refers to a leak in the membrane of the dialyzer.

Blood pressure: Pressure of the blood flowing through the blood vessels.

Blood vessel: Refers to either an artery or a vein.

Bone Marrow: The soft material filling the cavities of the bones where blood cells are produced.

BUN (blood urea nitrogen): A blood test that can determine the level of a certain waste product, urea, in the blood.

Cadaver donor: Term used for the nonliving, unrelated person whose kidney is used as a transplant organ for another person.

Calcitonin: A hormone secreted by the thyroid gland that protects against the loss of minerals in the bones and counterbalances the effects of parathyroid and Vitamin D. The role of calcitonin in kidney failure is unclear.

Calcium: The most abundant element in the body, located in the bones and the teeth.

Continuous Ambulatory Peritoneal Dialysis (CAPD): A form of peritoneal dialysis in which the dialysate is in the peritoneum 24 hours a day, seven days a week.

Capillary dialyzer: A type of dialyzer consisting of thousands of tiny plastic tubes through which the patient's blood flows.

Cardiopulmonary Resuscitation (CPR): The coordinated set of treatments to restore cardiac (heart) and/or pulmonary (lung) function should either or both suddenly fail, as might happen from a heart attack, a drowning or electric shock.

Catheter: A plastic or rubber tube through which fluids enter or leave the body.

Continuous Cycling Peritoneal Dialysis (CCPD): A form of peritoneal dialysis that uses a machine and can be done at home.

Cell: A microscopic entity capable of performing all of the basic functions of life (moving, reproduction, etc.)

Chelation therapy: A form of treatment, using medication, for aluminum or iron overload.

Chloramines: A type of disinfectant used in some tap water that must be removed from water used in artificial kidney machines.

Chronic kidney failure: The slow destruction of normal kidney tissue that may occur over a period of months or years, and results in irreversible kidney damage requiring dialysis or transplantation.

Combined or comprehensive directive: An advance directive that includes both treatment and proxy preferences.

Competence (competency): The legal term for decision-making capacity, which requires 1) understanding of one's situation (diagnosis, prognosis); 2) ability to analyze risks and benefits of possible treatments as well as to understand the consequences of no treatment; and 3) the ability to make and state a choice or decision.

Creatinine: Creatinine, or creat, is a byproduct of normal muscle metabolism.

Cycler: The dialysis machine used in continuous cycling peritoneal dialysis (CCPD).

Decision-making capacity: The medical equivalent of the legal term competence, which is the ability to make health care decisions for oneself.

Dextrose: A sugar solution found in peritoneal dialysate that may also be added to the dialysate in hemodialysis.

Diabetes: A disease in which sugar is inadequately utilized due to a lack of insulin in the body or the body's inability to use normal amounts of insulin properly.

Diabetic nephropathy: Kidney failure resulting from diabetes when damaged blood vessels make the kidneys unable to filter the blood properly.

Dialysate: Dialysate or dialysate fluid is the solution used in dialysis to remove excess fluids and waste products from the blood.

Dialysis: Process of maintaining the chemical balance of the blood when the kidneys have failed. May refer to hemodialysis or peritoneal dialysis.

Dialysis dementia: A neurological disorder that may be caused by aluminum intoxication or high levels of aluminum in the body.

Dialyzer: That part of the hemodialysis system that contains the cellophane membrane through which blood passes during hemodialysis.

Diffusion: The method used during dialysis to remove waste products from the blood and to balance chemicals in the blood.

DNA: The material of cells that carries the genetic code.

Do Not Resuscitate (DNR) order: An order, written by a physician, to alert health care professionals to honor a patient's decision not to have cardiopulmonary resuscitation should a cardiac or pulmonary arrest occur.

Dose: The amount of a drug or therapy to be given at one time.

Dry weight: The weight at which the body's blood pressure is normal and no swelling is present (all excess fluid is removed).

Durable Power of Attorney for Health Care (DBAHC): A written document (advance directive) that appoints another individual (or successor individuals) as proxy or surrogate to make health care decisions on behalf of the person or principal. This appointment becomes effective only upon the principal's loss of ability to make decisions for him- or herself.

Edema: Swelling in a specific area of the body due to a retention of excess fluids.

Electrocardiogram: Electrocardiogram, or EKG, is a tracing of the electrical rhythm of the heart, which is made by an instrument called an electrocardiograph.

Enzyme: A substance manufactured by tissue in the body, such as the liver or heart, that stimulates chemical changes.

EPO: The abbreviation for erythropoietin or recombinant human erythropoietin (here EPO is used to mean recombinant human erythropoietin).

Erythropoietin: A hormone that is released by functioning kidneys that helps the bone marrow to make red blood cells.

End-stage renal disease (ESRD): ESRD has the same meaning as the term chronic kidney failure, or that stage of kidney damage that requires dialysis or kidney transplantation.

Express (expressed) wishes: Health care preferences stated clearly by an individual as those he or she would or would not want under specific circumstances.

Fistula: An access method consisting of a surgically prepared, direct internal connection between an artery and a vein.

Fluid overload: Refers to a condition in which excess sodium and fluid build up in the body between dialysis treatments.

Folic acid: A substance necessary for red blood cell production.

Full-care facility: An outpatient dialysis center, which may or may not be based in a hospital.

Gene: A unit of DNA that carries the special genetic code necessary to determine an attribute of a cell or organism.

Genetic Code: The information of cells that tell cells what functions they will perform, how they will grow, and what they will produce. Altogether, the genetic code determines what characteristics an organism (such as a human being) will have (such as eye color or height).

Glomerulonephritis: A disease involving an inflammation in the tissues of the kidney and that destroys the kidney tissues.

Graft: An internal access device using synthetic material to surgically connect an artery to a vein.

Gram: A unit of weight in the metric system.

Hematocrit: A measure of the amount of red blood cells in the body.

Hemo: Means blood.

Hemodialysis: A form of dialysis that uses an artificial kidney machine to remove fluids and waste products from the bloodstream.

Hemoglobin: The oxygen-carrying pigment of red blood cells; what makes red blood cells red.

Heparin: A substance given to prevent blood from clotting.

Hepatitis: A viral infection of the liver.

Hepatitis A (infectious hepatitis): Can be contracted through close contact with an infected individual. Generally short-lived, and generally results in complete recovery.

Hepatitis B (serum hepatitis): A type of hepatitis transmitted through blood, intimate contact with an infected individual, IV drug abuse and also from an infected mother to the baby in the uterus. Many people develop chronic illness from hepatitis B, which can cause liver damage, and even liver cancer. Vaccination against hepatitis B is available and recommended for patients with kidney disease.

Hepatitis B Antigen Test: A test that determines the presence of an antigen associated with a type of hepatitis (serum hepatitis).

Hepatitis C: A form of chronic hepatitis, usually transmitted through blood transfusions or contaminated needles.

High-flux hemodialysis: A dialysis technique that speeds up the dialysis process.

Home dialysis: Self-care dialysis at home.

Hormones: Substances released by glands in the body to stimulate an activity elsewhere in the body.

Hyperkalemia: A condition in which high levels of potassium build up in the blood.

Hypertension: High blood pressure.

Hypotension: Abnormally low blood pressure.

Immunosuppressive drugs: Medications that help to prevent the rejection of transplanted organs, such as kidneys.

Incompetence (incompetency): In the broad sense, a lack of decision-making capacity, but in the narrow or legal sense, either a lack of decision-making ability determined by a court or not yet having reached the age of majority that legally entitles an individual to make decisions for him- or herself.

Informed consent (or refusal): The legal right to make health care decisions for oneself (and to be provided the information necessary to do so).

IPD (intermittent peritoneal dialysis): A form of peritoneal dialysis that requires a machine to perform the exchanges and is usually done in a hospital or clinic.

Insulin: The hormone produced in the pancreas and used by the tissues to get energy from blood sugar.

Iron: A metallic element found in hemoglobin.

Kidney: One of two organs located in the middle of the back, one on each side of the spine. Their function is to maintain the chemical balance of the body.

Kidney donor: The person from whom a healthy kidney is taken to be transplanted into another person.

Kidney transplantation: The removal of a kidney from either a living relative of the patient or from an unrelated, usually deceased, person, and surgically placing the new kidney into the person with kidney failure.

Living will: An advance directive of the treatment directive type, but usually limiting treatment that one would wish. It is a written statement made by one who is competent regarding his preference for treatment or treatment limitation should specific circumstances develop and should the individual at that time be incapable of making health care decisions for him- or herself.

MediCaid: A federal-state supported program to pay for health care for needy and low-income residents.

MediCal: MediCaid in California.

Medicare: Government-provided medical insurance under the Social Security Act.

Natural Death Act: Legislation allowing one to direct his or her physician to withhold or withdraw life-sustaining treatment (and thereby to allow a natural death) in the event of terminal illness, sometimes with the additional requirement of disability or infirmity.

Nephrectomy: Surgical removal of a kidney.

Nephrologist: Refers to a physician who is an internist primarily concerned with the medical treatment of patients with kidney disease or kidney failure.

Nephrology: Scientific study of the kidney.

Nephron: A tiny filter that is part of the kidney's structure and acts to maintain the body's chemical balance.

Neuropathy: Refers to any disease of the nerves that may cause nerve injury and a change in feeling in the feet, legs or hands.

Organism: A living thing made up of many cells.

Parallel flow dialyzer: A type of dialyzer consisting of layers of membrane arranged one on top of the other.

Parathyroid gland: One of several small glands located in the neck that releases a hormone that regulates the calcium and phosphorus level in the blood.

Patient Self Determination Act (PSDA): A federal statute requiring hospitals, long-term care facilities, hospice programs, home health agencies and prepaid health plans to provide patients with information about their rights to accept or refuse treatment and to formulate advance directives.

Peritoneal dialysis (PD): A form of dialysis similar in principle to hemodialysis. However, instead of using a dialyzer as in hemodialysis, the lining of the patient's abdominal cavity, or the peritoneum, is used.

Peritoneum: The membrane lining of the abdominal cavity.

Peritonitis: Refers to an infection inside the abdominal cavity and is associated with peritoneal dialysis.

Phosphate binders: Medication given to prevent the phosphorus in food from being absorbed in the body.

Phosphorus: An important element of the body which, when combined with calcium, helps to form bones. Excess levels of phosphorus, however, can rob the bones of needed calcium.

Pigment: Any organic coloring matter (for example, the color of red blood cells, hair, eyes, etc.).

Polycystic kidney disease: A hereditary disease that causes the normal kidney tissue to be replaced by cysts.

Potassium: A mineral needed by the body for normal heart and muscle function. Excess potassium in the body, or hyperkalemia, may be harmful.

Proxy: A word interchangeable with surrogate, indicating a person authorized or appointed to act for another individual.

Proxy directive: Names the individual or successor individuals who are to make health care decisions for a patient should he or she become unable to make or state decisions.

Pyelonephritis: A disease often caused by a bacterial infection of the kidneys.

Recombinant DNA Technology: The process of placing different genes into a cell to change the genetic make-up of the cell; it will alter the cell so that the cell will do things it would not do otherwise (like make large amounts of EPO).

Recombinant Human Erythropoietin: A hormone made through biotechnology that is very similar to the natural hormone (erythropoietin), which stimulates the production of red blood cells in the bone marrow.

Red blood cells: The oxygen-carrying cells of the bloodstream.

Rejection: The body's means of destroying the presence of a foreign substance or tissues from an outside source.

Renal: Refers to the kidney.

Renal ateriogram: X-ray of the arteries of the kidney.

Renin: A hormone that helps to control blood pressure. In nonfunctioning kidneys, the release of renin can become uncontrollable and can cause high blood pressure.

Saline: A salt solution containing sodium and chloride.

Satellite dialysis center: A dialysis center that is located outside of a hospital (also known as a "free-standing" dialysis center).

Self-care dialysis: Involves the patient being responsible for most of his or her own care with the assistance of another trained individual.

Sodium: A mineral found in the body that helps regulate the fluid content in the body.

Substituted judgment: An educated guess about what health care an individual would want based upon statements he or she

174

had made previously or upon knowledge of his or her values, beliefs or attitudes.

Success rate: Refers to successful kidney transplantation in which the kidney function is maintained for a sufficient length of time, usually at least a year.

Surrogate: A term interchangeable with proxy and indicating a person authorized or appointed to act for another.

Tissue typing: A laboratory procedure used to determine the degree of compatibility between the donor kidney and the recipient of the kidney transplant.

Toxins: Waste products in the blood or any substance that is toxic to the body.

Transfusion: The injection of fluid, especially blood or plasma, into a vein.

Treatment directive or instruction directive: An advance directive indicating treatment one would want and/or treatment one would not want, usually with some specification of the circumstances under which one would want or not want the treatment.

Ultrafiltration: The method used to remove excess fluids from the blood during dialysis.

Unit: A standard of measure, weight or any other quantity.

Uremia: A condition associated with the loss of kidney function and the buildup of waste products in the blood.

Ureter: The tube that carries urine from the kidney to the bladder.

Urethra: The tube that carries urine from the bladder to the outside of the body.

Urologist: A surgeon primarily concerned with the diagnosis and surgical treatment of disorders of the urinary system. Some urologists are also involved with transplant surgery.

Values History: A series of questions intended to elicit the beliefs, values, health and treatment preferences of an individual.

Vein: A vessel carrying blood to the heart.

Vitamin: An organic substance that occurs in natural foods and is necessary in trace amounts for normal metabolic functioning of the body.

Vitamin A: A fat-soluble vitamin found in egg yolk, fish-liver oils, liver, butter, cheese and many vegetables.

Vitamin B Complex: An important group of water-soluble vitamins isolated from liver, yeast and other sources that includes thiamin, riboflavin, niacin, niacinimide, the vitamin B6 group, biotin, pantothenic acid, folic acid and others. The vitamin B complex group affects growth, appetite, lactation and the gastrointestinal, nervous and endocrine systems.

Vitamin B12: Found primarily in animal products; essential for red blood cell formation.

Vitamin C: Ascorbic acid, found in citrus fruits and vegetables; aids in growth and prevents diseases such as scurvy.

Vitamin D: A fat-soluble vitamin found in milk products and from exposure to sunlight; necessary for the absorption of calcium and phosphorous; valuable in the formation of bones and teeth.

Vitamin E: A fat-soluble vitamin necessary in the body for reproduction and muscular development that is found in whole grains and vegetables.

Vitamin K: Found in green vegetables; important for the normal clotting of blood.

White blood cells: Blood cells in the body that destroy bacteria and foreign matter in the bloodstream.

BIBLIOGRAPHY

Contemporary Dialysis and Nephrology, "ESRD Provisions of the Sixth Omnibus Budget Reconciliation Act of 1986," *Contemporary Dialysis and Nephrology*, p. 43-45, December, 1986.

Denton, Sherwood E., *A Search for Answers*, Arizona Kidney Foundation, Phoenix, AZ, 1976.

Dialysis and Transplantation, "Access Device in CAPD Patients," *Dialysis and Transplantation*, vol. 15, no. 9, p. 487, September, 1986.

Dialysis and Transplantation, "Use of Orthoclone OKT3 Monoclonal Antibody for Acute Allograft Rejection," *Dialysis and Transplantation*, vol. 15, no. 9, p. 4-84, September, 1986.

Faber, Richard L., Kidney Patient handbook, Kidney Transplant/ Dialysis Association, Inc., Boston, MA, 1979.

Galonsky, B.S., R., Hutchisson, J., and Friedman, M.D., E., "Research and Technology — Have Kidney - Will Travel," *NAPHT NEWS*, p. 30, February, 1983.

Glabman, Sheldon, *Your Kidneys, Their Care and Their Cure*, E.P. Dutton & Co., Inc., New York City, NY, 1976.

Hathaway, David S., *Living with End Stage Renal Disease*, U.S. Department of Health, Education, and Welfare, Washington D.C., 1976.

Iowa Council of Renal Nutritionists, *Dietary Considerations in Renal Disease*, National Kidney Foundation of Iowa, Des Moines, IA, 1979.

Los Angeles District of the California Dietetic Association, *A Guide to Protein Controlled Diets for Dietitans*, Los Angeles District of the California Dietetic Association, Los Angeles, CA, 1977.

Medical World News, "Hepatitis B Vaccine No Longer Doubtful," *Medical World News*, p. 68, August, 1986.

L.A. Metropolitan Water District, *Chloramines and Your Water*, Metropolitan Water District, Los Angeles, CA, 1984.

National Kidney Foundation of Middle Tennessee, "Aluminum Intoxication," Kidney Foundation Newsletter, Spring/Summer, 1986.

National Kidney Foundation of Southern California, *A Guide to Traveling for People Receiving Dialysis Treatment*, National Kidney Foundation of Southern California, Los Angeles, CA, 1980.

National Kidney Foundation of Southern California, *Resources for People Receiving Dialysis Treatment*, National Kidney Foundation of Southern California, Los Angeles, CA, 1980.

Oberley, E., Painter, P., and Sacksteder, P., *Fitness After Kidney Failure*, National Kidney Foundation, New York City, NY, 1985.

Oberley, Edith T. and Terry D. Oberley, *Understanding Your New Life with Dialysis*, Charles C. Thomas, Springfield, IL, 1979.

Peirce, John C., *Diet Instruction Manual*, National Kidney Foundation of Michigan, Ann Arbor, MI, 1975.

Renalife, "AIDS and Kidney Patients: Guidelines for Protection," *Renalife*, March/April, 1986.

Richards, Carl J., *Understanding How Fellow Patients Cope*, National Kidney Foundation of Iowa, Des Moines, IA, 1977.

Richards, Carl J., *Understanding Your Dialysis*, National Kidney Foundation of Iowa, Des Moines, IA, 1977.

Richards, Carl J., *Understanding Your Renal Diet*, National Kidney Foundation of Iowa, Des Moines, IA, 1977.

U.S. Department of Health, Education, and Welfare, *Medicare Coverage of Kidney Dialysis and Transplant Services*, U.S. Department of Health, Education, and Welfare, Washington, D.C., 1980.

National Association of Patients on Hemodialysis and Transplantation, NAPHT — *The Voice of the Kidney Patient*, NAPHT, Great Neck, NY, 1980.

National Kidney Foundation, *Basic Information for Prospective Kidney Donors*, National Kidney Foundation, New York City, NY, 1978.

National Kidney Foundation, CAPD: *A New Alternative in Dialysis*, National Kidney Foundation, New York City, NY, 1980.

National Kidney Foundation, *Diabetes and Kidney Disease*, National Kidney Foundation, New York City, NY, 1986.

National Kidney Foundation, *Dialysis*, National Kidney Foundation, New York City, NY, 1985.

National Kidney Foundation, *Nutrition and Changing Kidney Function*, National Kidney Foundation, New York City, NY, 1986.

National Kidney Foundation, *Nutrition and Peritoneal Dialysis*, National Kidney Foundation, New York City, NY, 1986.

National Kidney Foundation, *Peritoneal Dialysis*, National Kidney Foundation, New York City, NY, 1986.

National Kidney Foundation, *Polycystic Kidney Disease*, National Kidney Foundation, New York City, NY, 1986.

National Kidney Foundation, *Social Work Services for the Patient with Chronic Renal Failure*, National Kidney Foundation, New York City, NY, 1978.

National Kidney Foundation, *The Artificial Kidney Machine. When You Need It. How it Works.*, National Kidney Foundation, New York City, NY, 1979.

National Kidney Foundation, *Transplantation*, National Kidney Foundation, New York City, NY, 1986.

APPENDICES

APPENDIX A
BLOOD TESTS

Abbreviation	Type of Test	Reason for Test
Al	Aluminum	A trace metal. High levels suggest aluminum intoxication and may require chelation therapy, which may cause brain dysfunction or bone disease.
Alb.	Albumin	Protein substance that helps hold fluid in blood vessels.
Alk Phos	Alkaline Phosphatase	An enzyme (a type of protein) in the liver and in bone; elevated levels may indicate liver or bone disease.
BUN	Blood Urea Nitrogen	Urea; byproduct of protein metabolism, indicator of levels of waste products in the blood, diet protein intake and the effectiveness of dialysis.
Ca	Calcium	Needed for bone-building; abnormal levels may be due to too much or too little calcium being deposited in bones or being absorbed from the diet.
Chol	Cholesterol	Fatty substance in blood; abnormal levels may lead to heart and blood vessel disease. Low levels indicate malnutrition.
Cl	Chloride	An essential element of blood that rises when bicarbonate falls.

Creat or Cr	Creatinine	Another indicator of toxin levels, which is related to the effectiveness of removal by the kidneys and dialysis and to one's muscle mass (rather than dietary intake).
Fe	Iron	Needed for red blood cells to be produced normally and to carry oxygen.
Ferritin	——	A protein that binds iron in the body. Low levels indicate a need for iron therapy. High levels occur when there is an excess of iron in the body, but also when there is an acute inflammation in the body.
Glu	Glucose	Blood sugar, which is high in diabetics, and most commonly is low when too much medication (insulin or oral hypoglycemic) is given to a diabetic.
HB$_S$ Ag	Hepatitis B Surface Antigen	Test for current infection with (serum) Hepatitis B and for contagiousness.
HB$_S$AS	Hepatitis B Surface Antibody	Test for current or prior infection with Hepatitis B.
HC03	Bicarbonate	A base, and, thus, indirectly, a test of acidity in the blood.
Hct	Hematocrit	Percentage of the blood that is red blood cells; low levels indicate anemia.
Hgb	Hemoglobin	The molecule within RBCs, which contains iron and which transports the oxygen and carbon dioxide. A low level indicates anemia and/or iron deficiency.

$1,25(OH)_2, D_3$	Calcitriol	The active form of Vitamin D (activated by the liver and by the kidneys), which has also been produced by pharmaceutical firms to be used as a medication.
K	Potassium	An essential element of the blood and especially of the fluid inside cells; abnormal levels (both high and low) could adversely affect the heart and cause muscle weakness.
LDH	Lactic Dehydrogenase	An enzyme; elevations may indicate general muscle damage, or increased destruction of red blood cells.
Mg	Magnesium	An element similar to calcium, which is predominantly inside cells and important to their function.
Na	Sodium	An essential element of blood and of the fluid outside cells; lower levels can cause muscle cramping; high levels cause excessive thirst, and lead to edema and hypertension.
P or PO_4	Phosphate	Elevated levels indicate excessive intake or failure to comply with phosphate binding medications or excessive parathyroid hormone.
Plts	Platelets	Small cells in the blood that help the blood to clot.
PTH	Parathyroid Hormone	A hormone produced in the parathyroid glands. High levels may cause bone disease.

RBC	Red Blood Cells or Erythrocytes	The number of red blood cells that carry oxygen to the tissues and carbon dioxide from the tissues to the lungs. Normally, RBCs have a life span of 120 days.
Retics	Reticulocytes	Young, red blood cells. If a high percentage of red blood cells are reticulocytes, this is evidence of active red blood cell formation.
SGOT	Serum Glutamic Oxalocetic Transaminase	An enzyme; elevations usually indicate liver damage, though this enzyme also rises acutely if there is muscle injury, as in a heart attack.
SGPT	Serum	An enzyme; elevations indicate liver damage.
T. Bili.	Total Bilirubin	Waste product which must be removed by liver through the bile ducts and increases with liver or gall bladder disease.
T.P.	Total Protein	Amount of protein in blood, mostly albumin and globulin.
Transferrin	Transferrin	A protein that transports iron in the blood (before it is incorporated in Hgb) and that increases when iron is deficient.
Uric Acid	Uric Acid	A waste product from protein in the diet that should be removed to prevent gouty arthritis and kidney stones.
WBC	White Blood Cells	Cells that fight infection. High levels usually indicate infection, and very low levels indicate susceptibility to infection.

From *Understanding Your New Life With Dialysis*, Edith T. Oberley, M.A., and Terry D. Oberley, M.D., Ph.D., second edition, 1978. Courtesy of Charles C Thomas, Publisher, Springfield, Illinois.

APPENDIX B
FOOD LISTS

Foods are grouped under the following main headings: meats and meat substitutes, dairy products, breads and cereals, fruits, vegetables and miscellaneous. An average nutrient value of protein, sodium, potassium and calories has been established for each group.

ABBREVIATIONS

c	= cup	K	= potassium	
CA	= calcium	lge	= large	
CAL	= calories	Low Sod	= Low Sodium	
CHO	= carbohydrate	med	= medium	
ck	= cooked	mEq	= milliequivalent	
cnd	= canned	mg	= milligram	
diam	= diameter	NA	= sodium	
froz	= frozen	oz	= ounce	
gm	= gram	P	= phosphorus	

PRO	= protein
sm	= small
sw	= sweetened
	(canned in syrup)
Tbsp	= tablespoon
tsp	= teaspoon
tr	= trace
unsw	= unsweetened
"	= inch

LOW SODIUM PROTEIN LIST

AVERAGES: Calories: 60 Protein: 8 gm Sodium: 30 mg Potassium: 100 mg Calcium: 10 mg Phosphorus: 70 mg

FOOD ITEM	HOUSEHOLD MEASURE	gm	CAL	gm PRO	m FAT	gm CHO	mg CA	mg P	mg NA	mg K
Beef brisket	1 oz.	28	68	8	4	0	2	61	20	96
Beef chuck roast	1 oz.	28	66	9	3	0	2	76	19	82
Beef rib roast	1 oz.	28	65	7	4	0	3	57	20	108
Beef round	1 oz.	28	55	8	2	0	2	67	18	117
Beef loin	1 oz.	28	57	8	2	0	2	62	19	112
Beef, ground, x-lean	1 oz.	28	72	7	5	1	2	46	20	89
Cottage cheese, dry	1/4 c.	36	31	6	trace	0	12	38	5	12
Chicken, no skin	1 oz.	28	53	8	2	0	4	55	24	68
Chicken, canned LS	1 oz.	28	59	8	4	0	4	55	14	44
Duck, no skin	1 oz.	28	56	7	3	0	3	57	18	70
Egg, whole	1 lg	50	79	6	6	trace	28	90	69	65
Egg whites	2	66	32	7	trace	trace	8	8	100	90
Lamb	1 oz.	8	56	8	2	0	4	65	20	88
Pork, fresh	1 oz.	28	66	8	4	0	2	73	20	103
Rabbit	1 oz.	28	62	8	3	0	6	74	12	105
Turkey, no skin	1 oz.	28	42	8	1	0	5	58	19	74
Veal	1 oz.	28	68	8	4	0	3	61	18	80
Venison	1 oz.	28	42	8	1	0	6	75	20	96

LOW SODIUM PROTEIN LIST (continued)

AVERAGES: Calories: 60 Protein: 8 gm Sodium: 30 mg Potassium: 100 mg Calcium: 10 mg Phosphorus: 70 mg

FOOD ITEM	HOUSEHOLD MEASURE	gm	CAL	gm PRO	m FAT	gm CHO	mg CA	mg P	mg NA	mg K
ORGAN MEATS:										
Beef heart	1 oz.	28	49	8	2	trace	1	71	18	66
Beef kidney	1 oz.	28	41	7	1	trace	5	87	38	51
Beef liver	1 oz.	28	61	8	2	2	3	131	30	103
Beef tongue	1 oz.	28	80	6	6	trace	2	40	17	51
Chicken gizzard	1/4 c.	36	55	10	1	trace	4	56	24	65
Chicken liver	1/4 c.	35	55	9	2	trace	5	109	18	49
Pork liver	1 oz.	28	47	7	1	1	3	68	14	43
Turkey giblets	1/4 c.	36	61	10	2	1	4	74	21	73
SEAFOOD:										
Bass, baked	1 oz.	28	69	6	5	1	23	64	16	61
Clams, steamed	3 med.	42	38	6	2	2	20	96	24	131
Cod, broiled	1 oz.	28	48	8	2	0	9	78	31	113
Haddock, broiled	1 oz.	8	39	6	2	trace	4	64	20	100
Salmon, Sole/Flounder, broiled	1 oz.	28	55	8	2	0	10	98	38	146
Halibut	1 oz.	28	40	8	1	0	17	80	20	163
Lobster	1/4 c.	36	35	7	1	trace	24	69	76	65
Oysters, raw	3 med.	57	68	7	2	4	37	126	90	181
Scallops, steamed	3 lg.	28	31	7	trace	1	10	86	75	141
Shrimp, boiled	5 lg.	28	31	7	trace	0	91	76	51	113
Tuna, canned LS	1/4 c.	40	51	11	1	0	2	89	16	105

HIGH SODIUM PROTEIN LIST

AVERAGES: Calories: 60 Protein: 8 gm Sodium: 180 mg Potassium: 100 mg Calcium: 20 mg Phosphorus: 80 mg

FOOD ITEM	HOUSEHOLD MEASURE	gm	CAL	gm PRO	m FAT	gm CHO	mg CA	mg P	mg NA	mg K
Chicken, canned	1 oz.	28	47	6	2	0	4	50	14	339
Cottage cheese, reg.	1/4 c.	56	58	7	2	2	34	74	228	48
Cottage cheese, LF	1/4 c.	56	51	8	1	2	38	85	120	128
Salmon, canned-oil	1/4 c.	40	62	8	3	0	90	120	180	140
Tuna, canned-oil	1/4 c.	40	84	11	5	trace	3	93	224	104
Tuna, canned-water	1/4 c.	40	48	11	1	trace	3	82	177	110
Turkey breast, smkd.	1 oz.	28	35	6	1	trace	1	80	227	69
Turkey, canned	1 oz.	28	46	7	2	0	3	58	133	74
Turkey roll	1 oz.	28	42	5	2	trace	9	48	166	77

SUPPLEMENTAL PROTEIN LIST

Directions for use: These foods contribute a significant amount of potassium and phosphorus and are sources of low biological value protein, and should be calculated into a Patient diet on an individual basis.

AVERAGES: Calories: 120 Protein: 8 gm Sodium: 10 mg Potassium: 30 mg Calcium: 35 mg Phosphorus: 130 mg

FOOD ITEM	HOUSEHOLD MEASURE	gm	CAL	gm PRO	m FAT	gm CHO	mg CA	mg P	mg NA	mg K
Beans, cooked without salt:										
Blackeyed peas	1/2 c.	28	47	6	2	0	4	50	14	339
Garbanzo beans	1/2 c.	56	58	7	2	2	34	74	228	48
Kidney beans	1/2 c.	56	51	8	1	2	38	85	120	128
Lentils	2/3 c.	40	62	8	3	0	90	120	180	140
Peanut butter*	2 Tbs.	40	84	11	5	trace	3	93	224	104
*unsalted										

DAIRY LIST

AVERAGES: Calories: Varies Protein: 4 gm Sodium: 85 mg Potassium: 190 mg Calcium: 150 mg Phosphorus: 120 mg

FOOD ITEM	HOUSEHOLD MEASURE	gm	CAL.	gm PRO	m FAT	gm CHO	mg CA	mg P	mg NA	mg K
MILK:										
Whole milk	1/2 c.	122	75	4	4	6	146	114	60	185
LF milk, 2%	1/2 c.	122	60	4	2	6	148	116	61	188
LF milk, hi pro	1/2 c.	123	68	5	2	7	176	138	72	224
Non-fat milk	1/2 c.	122	43	4	trace	6	151	124	63	203
Buttermilk	1/2 c.	122	50	4	1	6	142	110	128	166
Calci-milk	1/2 c.	122	45	4	trace	6	200	118	62	190
Choc. milk, whole	1/2 c.	125	104	4	4	13	140	126	74	208
Choc. milk, LF	1/2 c.	125	90	4	2	13	142	127	75	211
Cocoa, mix + water	1 c.	240	110	4	3	20	107	108	154	176
Cream, half & half	1/2 c.	120	158	4	14	5	127	115	49	157
Eggnog, no ETOH	1/2 c.	127	171	5	10	17	165	139	69	210
Evap. milk, whole	1/4 c.	63	84	4	5	6	164	128	66	191
Evap. milk, skim	1/4 c.	64	50	5	trace	7	184	124	74	212
Goat's milk, skim	1/2 c.	122	84	5	5	6	163	135	61	250
LactAid, LF	1/2 c.	122	60	4	2	6	120	118	62	190
LactAid, skim	1/2 c.	122	45	4	trace	6	120	96	62	190
Powd/dry NF milk	2 Tbs.	15	54	5	trace	8	188	145	80	269

DAIRY LIST (continued)

AVERAGES: Calories: Varies Protein: 4 gm Sodium: 85 mg Potassium: 190 mg Calcium: 150 mg Phosphorus: 120 mg

FOOD ITEM	HOUSEHOLD MEASURE	gm	CAL	gm PRO	m FAT	gm CHO	mg CA	mg P	mg NA	mg K
PUDDING:										
D'zerta, w/skim	1/2 c.	150	67	4	0	12	120	100	67	190
Mix, not instant	1/2 c.	130	160	4	4	30	132	123	167	190
Cup, Swiss Miss	4 oz.	113	150	3	6	24	80	80	180	190
Pudd. pop, Jello	2 bars	108	150	4	4	26	128	64	130	190
YOGURT:										
LF, fruited	1/2 c.	113	116	6	1	22	172	135	66	221
LF, vanilla	1/2 c.	113	97	6	1	16	194	153	75	249
LF, plain	1/2 c.	133	72	6	2	8	207	163	80	265
Non-fat, plain	1/2 c.	114	58	6	trace	8	178	134	64	142
FROZEN DESSERTS:										
Fudgsicle	1 bar	73	91	4	trace	19	129	99	55	173
Ice cream, no nuts	3/4 c.	105	232	3	15	24	122	93	84	180
Ice milk, hard	3/4 c.	100	138	4	4	22	132	97	79	199
Soft-serve ice milk	1/2 c.	88	112	4	2	19	137	101	82	206

CHEESE LIST

AVERAGES: Calories: Varies Protein: 4 gm Sodium: 85 mg Potassium: 190 mg Calcium: 150 mg Phosphorus: 120 mg

FOOD ITEM	HOUSEHOLD MEASURE	gm	CAL	gm PRO	m FAT	gm CHO	mg CA	mg P	mg NA	mg K
NATURAL CHEESES:										
Bleu cheese	1/2 oz.	14	50	3	4	trace	75	55	198	36
Brie cheese	1/2 oz.	14	48	3	4	0	26	26	89	22
Cheddar cheese	1/2 oz.	14	57	4	4	0	102	72	88	14
Gouda cheese	1/2 oz.	14	50	4	4	trace	99	78	116	17
Colby cheese	1/2 oz.	14	56	3	4	trace	97	64	86	18
Gruyere cheese	1/2 oz.	14	58	4	4	0	144	86	48	12
Jack cheese	1/2 oz.	14	53	3	4	0	106	63	76	12
Mozzarella, skim	1/2 oz.	14	36	3	2	0	92	66	66	12
Swiss cheese	1/2 oz.	14	54	4	4	trace	136	86	37	16

SUPPLEMENTAL DAIRY LIST

Directions for use: These foods contribute a significant amount of sodium, potassium and phosphorus, and should be calculated into patient's diet on an individual basis.

AVERAGES: Calories: Varies Protein: 6 gm Sodium: 165 mg Potassium: 400 mg Calcium: 260 mg Phosphorus: 200 mg

FOOD ITEM	HOUSEHOLD MEASURE	gm	CAL	gm PRO	m FAT	gm CHO	mg CA	mg P	mg NA	mg K
Alba 66 cocoa	1 pkt.	—	60	5	trace	10	320	240	180	425
Alba 77 frosty	1 pkt.	—	70	6	1	11	310	180	190	430
Custard from mix	1/2 c.	143	161	5	5	23	174	174	219	254
Instant Breakfast:										
1 pkt. + whole milk	1/2 c.	265	280	15	9	34	378	378	285	687
Ovaltine + milk	1/2 c.	132	114	5	4	15	151	151	114	300
Low sodium milk	1/2 c.	122	74	4	4	5	104	104	3	308

REGULAR BREAD AND STARCH LIST

AVERAGES: Calories: 90 Protein: 2 gm Sodium: 160 mg Potassium: 35 mg Calcium: 20 mg Phosphorus: 35 mg

FOOD ITEM	HOUSEHOLD MEASURE	gm	CAL	gm PRO	m FAT	gm CHO	mg CA	mg P	mg NA	mg K
BREADS:										
Cracked wheat	1 sl.	25	66	2	trace	13	22	32	132	34
French	1 sl.	15	44	1	trace	8	6	13	87	14
Vienna	1 sl.	25	73	2	trace	14	11	21	145	23
Raisin	1 sl.	25	66	2	trace	13	18	22	91	58
Rye	1 sl.	25	61	2	trace	13	19	37	139	36
White	1 sl.	28	76	2	trace	14	24	27	142	39
Whole wheat	1 sl.	28	56	2	trace	11	23	52	121	63
Biscuit	1	28	97	2	4	14	31	64	225	30
Bread crumbs	1/2 c.	23	62	2	trace	11	22	23	112	27
Bread stuffing	1/4 c.	43	115	2	7	11	22	34	283	31
Bread sticks	2	12	46	1	trace	9	4	12	200	12
Blueberry muffin	1	40	122	3	4	17	34	53	253	46
Corn muffin	1	40	126	3	4	19	42	68	192	54
Cornbread	2" x 2"	25	53	2	2	8	29	47	150	39
Pancake	1 (4")	27	62	2	2	9	42	54	134	38
Roll, brn/serve	1	28	92	2	2	15	14	25	157	28
Roll, cloverleaf	1	35	119	3	3	20	16	36	98	41
Roll, hamburger	1/2	20	57	2	1	10	27	17	121	19
Roll, hard	1	25	78	3	trace	15	12	23	156	24
Roll, hot dog	1/2	40	118	4	2	21	30	34	202	38

REGULAR BREAD AND STARCH LIST (continued)

AVERAGES: Calories: 90 Protein: 2 gm Sodium: 160 mg Potassium: 35 mg Calcium: 20 mg Phosphorus: 35 mg

FOOD ITEM	HOUSEHOLD MEASURE	gm	CAL	gm PRO	m FAT	gm CHO	mg CA	mg P	mg NA	mg K
Roll, parkerhouse	1	24	75	2	1	13	9	21	127	23
Tortilla, corn	1	30	67	2	1	13	42	55	53	53
Tortilla, flour	1 (6")	35	85	2	1	15	46	25	150	20
Taco shell	2	22	100	2	4	14	32	50	144	50
Waffle, frozen	1	28	71	2	2	12	34	59	181	45
Danish	1 sm.	38	165	3	9	18	20	43	143	44
Donut, cake	1	25	105	1	6	12	11	55	139	27
Donut, raised	1	30	124	2	8	11	11	23	70	24
DESSERTS:										
Cake, yellow	2" x 2"	48	175	2	6	28	40	67	107	43
Cake, pound	1 sl.	30	147	2	7	18	10	29	86	21
Cupcake, iced	1	42	152	2	5	25	40	60	118	43
Butter cookies	6	30	137	2	5	21	38	28	125	18
Choc chip cookies	2	21	101	1	5	14	8	22	77	26
Shortbread	4 pcs.	32	168	2	9	20	8	36	144	20
Sugar cookies	4	32	142	2	5	22	25	33	102	24
Sugar wafers	4	38	184	2	7	28	14	30	72	23
Vanilla wafers	10	35	152	2	6	21	14	22	88	26
Animal crackers	10	26	112	2	2	21	14	30	79	25

REGULAR BREAD AND STARCH LIST (continued)

AVERAGES: Calories: 90 Protein: 2 gm Sodium: 160 mg Potassium: 35 mg Calcium: 20 mg Phosphorus: 35 mg

FOOD ITEM	HOUSEHOLD MEASURE	gm	CAL	gm PRO	m FAT	gm CHO	mg CA	mg P	mg NA	mg K
Arrowroot crackers	6	30	141	2	5	22	18	39	72	33
Brownie	1 sm.	22	94	1	5	14	10	29	41	39
SNACKS:										
Fritos corn chips	1 oz.	28	155	2	10	16	29	47	183	38
Reg. tortilla chips	1 oz.	28	144	2	7	18	37	62	165	49
Saltines	8	23	98	2	3	16	5	21	250	27
Soda crackers	8	23	100	2	3	16	5	20	250	27
Oyster crackers	30	23	99	2	3	16	6	21	46	27
Ritz crackers	8	27	144	2	8	18	40	64	277	24
CEREALS:										
Captain Crunch	1 c.	35	146	2	3	28	11	47	243	49
Cocoa Krispies	1 c.	36	139	2	1	32	6	47	243	49
Corn Chex	1 c.	28	111	2	trace	25	3	11	271	23
Cornflakes	1 c.	26	100	2	trace	22	2	15	276	23
Fruity Pebbles	1 c.	32	131	1	2	28	3	19	179	24
Kix	1 c.	19	74	2	1	16	23	26	227	29
Rice Krispies	1 c.	28	112	2	trace	25	5	33	274	29
Sugar Frosted Flakes	1 c.	38	146	2	trace	34	3	15	238	21
Trix	1 c.	28	109	2	trace	25	6	19	181	27

LOW SODIUM BREAD AND STARCH LIST

AVERAGES: Calories: 90 Protein: 2 gm Sodium: 5 mg Potassium: 35 mg Calcium: 10 mg Phosphorus: 35 mg

FOOD ITEM	HOUSEHOLD MEASURE	gm	CAL	gm PRO	m FAT	gm CHO	mg CA	mg P	mg NA	mg K
BREADS:										
Rice wafers	2	18	70	2	0	16	—	—	20	50
Matzo	1 pc.	36	144	3	0	33	—	—	1	43
Low sod. bread	1 sl.	28	68	2	1	13	21	40	6	50
Ladyfingers	2	22	79	2	2	14	9	36	15	15
Melba tast	4 pcs.	20	60	2	1	11	—	—	12	36
Popcorn (no salt)	1 c.	14	54	2	1	11	2	39	0	28
Ice cream cone	1	45	45	1	trace	9	19	24	28	29
CEREALS: (Cooked without salt)										
Corn grits	1/2 c.	121	73	2	trace	16	1	15	0	27
Cream of rice	1/2 c.	122	63	1	trace	14	4	21	1	25
Cream of wheat	1/2 c.	124	72	2	trace	15	28	22	2	23
Farina	1/2 c.	117	58	2	trace	12	2	14	1	15
Oatmeal	1/2 c.	117	73	3	2	13	10	89	1	66
Malt-O-Meal	1/2 c.	121	62	2	trace	13	2	12	1	23
LS Cornflakes	1 c.	28	113	2	trace	25	12	14	3	21
LS Rice Krispies	1 c.	28	114	2	trace	26	19	29	3	22
Frosted MiniWheats	3 biscuits	22	77	2	trace	18	7	56	6	73
Puffed Rice	1 c.	15	57	1	trace	13	1	14	0	16

LOW SODIUM BREAD AND STARCH LIST (continued)

AVERAGES: Calories: 90 Protein: 2 gm Sodium: 5 mg Potassium: 35 mg Calcium: 10 mg Phosphorus: 35 mg

FOOD ITEM	HOUSEHOLD MEASURE	gm	CAL	gm PRO	m FAT	gm CHO	mg CA	mg P	mg NA	mg K
Puffed Wheat	1 c.	14	52	2	trace	11	4	50	1	49
Shredded Wheat	1 biscuit	24	83	3	trace	19	10	86	0	77
STARCHES: (Cooked without salt)										
Macaroni, cooked	1/2 c.	68	86	3	trace	18	8	39	0	47
Noodles, cooked	1/2 c.	80	102	3	1	18	8	47	2	35
Brown rice, cooked	1/2 c.	98	117	2	1	25	12	71	0	70
White rice, cooked	1/2 c.	73	112	2	trace	25	11	29	0	29
Spaghetti, cooked	1/2 c.	68	84	3	trace	18	7	39	1	47
White flour	2 Tbs.	16	57	2	trace	12	3	14	0	15

FRUIT LIST #1

AVERAGES: Calories: 60 Protein: <1 gm Sodium: 5 mg Potassium: 100 mg Calcium: 15 mg Phosphorus: 13 mg

FOOD ITEM	HOUSEHOLD MEASURE	gm	CAL	gm PRO	m FAT	gm CHO	mg CA	mg P	mg NA	mg K
FRUITS WITHOUT ADDED SUGAR:										
Acerola	10 ea.	48	20	trace	trace	4	10	10	3	70
Apple, dried	4 rings	26	62	trace	trace	17	4	10	22	115
Apple, fresh	1 sm.	69	41	trace	trace	11	5	5	0	80
Applesauce	1/2 c.	122	53	trace	trace	14	4	9	2	91
Blackberries	1/2 c.	74	43	1	trace	11	23	19	1	123
Blueberries	1/2 c.	75	40	trace	trace	10	5	8	3	53
Boysenberries	1/2 c.	122	44	1	trace	11	23	23	1	104
Carissa, fresh	2 ea.	40	24	trace	trace	5	4	2	2	104
Cherries, sour red, water-pack	1/2 c.	122	43	1	trace	11	13	12	9	120
Crabapples, sliced	1/2 c.	55	42	trace	trace	11	10	9	1	107
Cranberries, raw	1 c.	110	54	trace	trace	14	8	10	1	78
Fig, dried	1	19	48	1	trace	12	27	13	2	133
Fig, fresh	1	50	37	trace	trace	10	18	7	1	116
Fig, canned water	1/2 c.	124	65	1	trace	17	35	13	2	128
Fruit cocktail	1/2 c.	123	48	1	trace	13	8	16	5	117
Fruit salad, canned	1/2 c.	123	50	1	trace	13	11	15	6	120
Gooseberries	1/2 c.	75	34	1	trace	8	19	20	1	149
Grapes, fresh	1/2 c.	63	43	trace	trace	11	8	8	1	118
Kumquats	4 ea.	76	48	1	trace	12	32	16	4	148

FRUIT LIST #1 (continued)

AVERAGES: Calories: 60 Protein: <1 gm Sodium: 5 mg Potassium: 100 mg Calcium: 15 mg Phosphorus: 13 mg

FOOD ITEM	HOUSEHOLD MEASURE	gm	CAL	gm PRO	m FAT	gm CHO	mg CA	mg P	mg NA	mg K
Lemon, no peel	1 med.	58	17	1	trace	5	15	9	1	80
Lime, no peel	1 ea.	67	20	1	trace	7	22	12	1	68
Loganberries	1/2 c.	74	40	1	trace	10	19	19	1	107
Loquats, fresh	5 ea.	50	25	trace	trace	6	10	15	0	130
Lychees, fresh	8 ea.	77	48	1	trace	13	0	24	0	128
Mulberries	1/2 c.	70	31	1	trace	7	28	27	7	136
Oheloberries	1 c.	140	39	1	trace	10	10	14	2	54
Passion fruit	2 ea.	36	36	1	trace	8	4	24	10	126
Peaches, canned	1/2 c.	123	42	1	trace	11	5	17	5	140
Pears, canned	1/2 c.	123	49	trace	trace	13	8	12	4	92
Persimmon	1 ea.	25	32	trace	trace	8	7	7	0	78
Pineapple chunks	1/2 c.	124	57	1	trace	15	18	7	2	154
Pineapple, fresh	1/2 c.	78	39	trace	trace	10	6	6	1	88
Pitanga, fresh	1/2 c.	87	29	1	trace	6	8	10	3	89
Plum, fresh	1 med.	66	36	1	trace	9	2	7	0	113
Raspberries	1/2 c.	62	31	1	trace	7	14	8	0	94
Roselle, fresh	1 c.	57	28	1	trace	6	123	21	3	118
Strawberries	1/2 c.	75	24	trace	trace	6	11	12	1	117
Tamarind, fresh	10 ea.	20	50	trace	trace	13	10	20	10	130
Tangerine, fresh	1 med.	84	37	1	trace	9	12	8	1	132
Watermelon (1" sl.)	1/4 sl.	—	38	1	1	9	10	10	3	140

FRUIT LIST #1 (continued)

AVERAGES: Calories: 60 Protein: <1 gm Sodium: 5 mg Potassium: 100 mg Calcium: 15 mg Phosphorus: 13 mg

FOOD ITEM	HOUSEHOLD MEASURE	gm	CAL	gm PRO	m FAT	gm CHO	mg CA	mg P	mg NA	mg K
FRUIT JUICE - NO SUGAR ADDED:										
Acerola juice, fresh	1/2 c.	121	26	1	trace	6	12	11	4	118
Apple juice	1/2 c.	122	57	trace	trace	14	8	9	6	149
Lemon juice	1/2 c.	122	28	1	trace	9	11	9	13	138
Lime juice	1/2 c.	123	29	trace	trace	10	13	11	10	113

FRUIT LIST #2

AVERAGES: Calories: 60 Protein: <1 gm Sodium: 5 mg Potassium: 200 mg Calcium: 15 mg Phosphorus: 17 mg

FOOD ITEM	HOUSEHOLD MEASURE	gm	CAL	gm PRO	m FAT	gm CHO	mg CA	mg P	mg NA	mg K
FRUITS WITHOUT ADDED SUGAR:										
Apricot, fresh	2 ea.	71	34	1	trace	8	10	14	1	209
Apricot, canned	1/2 c.	123	46	1	trace	12	12	21	4	219
Apricot, dried	4 halves	14	34	1	trace	9	6	17	2	193
Carambola, fresh	1 ea.	127	42	1	trace	10	6	20	2	207
Cherries, sweet, fresh	1/2 c.	73	52	1	1	12	11	14	1	163
Cherries, sweet, canned	1/2 c.	125	63	1	trace	16	15	23	3	163
Dates, domestic	4 ea.	33	91	1	trace	24	11	13	1	216
Elderberries	1/2 c.	73	53	1	trace	13	28	29	0	203
Grapefruit, fresh	1/2	120	38	1	trace	10	14	10	0	167
Grapefruit, canned	1/2 c.	123	45	1	trace	11	19	14	6	185
Mandarin oranges	1/2 c.	124	46	1	0	12	14	13	7	165
Melonballs, frozen	1/2 c.	87	28	1	trace	7	9	11	27	242
Peach, fresh	1 sm.	87	37	1	trace	10	5	11	0	171
Pear, fresh	1 med.	166	98	1	1	25	19	18	1	208
Plum, canned	1/2 c.	125	62	1	trace	16	11	18	1	176
Prickly pear	1 ea.	103	42	1	trace	10	58	25	6	226
Prunes, dried	3 ea.	25	60	1	trace	16	13	20	1	188
Quince, fresh	1 ea.	92	53	trace	trace	14	10	16	4	181
Raisins	2 Tbs.	21	62	1	trace	16	10	20	2	155

FRUIT LIST #2 (continued)

AVERAGES: Calories: 60 Protein: <1 gm Sodium: 5 mg Potassium: 200 mg Calcium: 15 mg Phosphorus: 17 mg

FOOD ITEM	HOUSEHOLD MEASURE	gm	CAL	gm PRO	m FAT	gm CHO	mg CA	mg P	mg NA	mg K
FRUIT JUICE - NO SUGAR ADDED:										
Grapefruit juice	1/2 c.	124	49	1	trace	11	10	16	1	186
Orange juice	1/2 c.	124	55	1	trace	13	12	20	2	234
Orange-grapefruit juice	1/2 c.	124	54	1	trace	13	11	17	4	195
Pineapple juice	1/2 c.	125	68	1	trace	17	18	10	1	169

MISCELLANEOUS FRUIT LIST

Note: These fruits are very high in potassium and should be used only when approved by the dietitian.

FOOD ITEM	HOUSEHOLD MEASURE	gm	CAL	gm PRO	m FAT	gm CHO	mg CA	mg P	mg NA	mg K
Avocado	1/4	50	81	1	8	4	6	21	5	301
Banana	1 med.	114	105	1	1	27	7	22	1	451
Breadfruit, fresh	1/4 sm.	96	99	1	trace	26	17	29	2	470
Currants, dried	1/4 c.	36	102	2	trace	27	31	45	3	321
Guava, common	1 ea.	90	45	1	1	11	18	23	2	256
Kiwifruit, fresh	1 med.	76	46	1	trace	11	20	31	4	252
Mango, fresh	1 ea.	207	135	1	1	35	21	22	4	322
Melon, cantaloupe	1/4	134	47	1	trace	11	14	23	12	413
Melon, casaba	1/10	164	43	2	trace	10	8	11	20	344
Melon, honeydew	1/10	129	46	1	trace	12	8	13	13	350
Nectarine	1 ea.	136	67	1	1	16	6	22	0	288
Orange, fresh	1 sm.	159	64	2	1	25	111	35	3	312
Papaya, fresh	1/2 ea.	152	59	1	trace	15	36	8	4	390
Persimmon, dried	1 ea.	168	118	1	trace	31	13	28	3	270
Plantain, fresh	1/2 ea.	90	109	1	trace	29	3	31	4	447
Pomegranate, fresh	1	154	104	2	1	26	5	12	5	399
Prune juice, canned	1/2 c.	128	91	1	0	22	15	32	6	353
Prunes, canned	1/2 c.	117	123	1	trace	33	20	30	3	264
Pummelo, fresh	1/2 ea.	305	114	2	trace	29	12	51	4	659
Sapodilla, fresh	1 ea.	170	140	1	2	34	36	20	20	328
Soursop, fresh	1/2 ea.	313	208	3	1	53	44	85	44	870
Tamarind, pulp	1/2 c.	60	144	2	trace	38	45	68	17	377
Tangelo, fresh	1 med.	170	39	1	trace	9	27	20	2	296

VEGETABLE LIST #1

AVERAGES: Calories: 15 Protein: 1 gm Sodium: 20 mg Potassium: 100 mg Calcium: 20 mg Phosphorus: 18 mg

FOOD ITEM	HOUSEHOLD MEASURE	gm	CAL	gm PRO	m FAT	gm CHO	mg CA	mg P	mg NA	mg K
Amaranth, raw	1/2 c.	14	4	trace	trace	1	30	7	3	86
Bamboo shoots	1/2 c.	66	13	1	trace	2	5	17	5	52
Beans, Mung, raw	1/2 c.	52	16	2	trace	3	7	28	3	77
Beans, snap, raw	1/2 c.	55	17	1	trace	4	21	21	3	115
Beans, snap, cooked	1/2 c.	66	18	1	trace	4	26	18	4	112
Broccoli, raw	1/2 c.	44	12	1	trace	2	21	29	12	143
Cabbage, Chinese	1/2 c.	35	5	1	trace	1	37	13	23	88
Cabbage, green, raw	1/2 c.	35	8	trace	trace	2	16	8	6	86
Cabbage, red, raw	1/2 c.	35	10	1	trace	2	18	15	4	72
Carrots, cooked	1/2 c.	75	26	1	trace	6	21	20	42	141
Chicory root, raw	1/2 c.	45	33	1	trace	8	18	27	23	131
Cucumber, raw	1/2 c.	52	7	trace	trace	2	7	9	1	78
Dandelion, green, ckd	1/2 c.	52	17	1	trace	3	73	22	23	121
Eggplant, boiled	1/2 c.	48	13	trace	trace	3	3	11	2	119
Endive, raw	1/2 c.	25	4	trace	trace	1	13	7	6	79
Leeks, raw	1/2 c.	52	32	1	trace	7	39	18	10	94
Lettuce, iceberg	1/2 c.	60	9	1	trace	1	12	12	6	96
Lettuce, romaine	1/2 c.	28	4	1	trace	1	10	13	2	81
Mushrooms, raw	1/2 c.	35	9	1	trace	2	2	36	1	130
Mushroom, Shiitake	1/2 c.	73	40	1	trace	10	2	22	3	85
Mustard green, raw	1/2 c.	28	7	1	trace	1	29	12	7	99

VEGETABLE LIST #1 (continued)

AVERAGES: Calories: 15 Protein: 1 gm Sodium: 20 mg Potassium: 100 mg Calcium: 20 mg Phosphorus: 18 mg

FOOD ITEM	HOUSEHOLD MEASURE	gm	CAL	gm PRO	m FAT	gm CHO	mg CA	mg P	mg NA	mg K
Mustard green, cooked	1/2 c.	73	13	2	trace	2	64	24	15	123
Onions, raw	1/2 c.	80	27	1	trace	6	20	23	2	124
Pea pods, raw	1/2 c.	72	30	2	trace	5	31	38	3	144
Peas & Carrots, cooked	1/2 c.	80	38	3	trace	8	18	39	55	127
Pepper, sweet, raw	1/2 c.	50	12	trace	trace	3	3	11	2	98
Purslane, raw	1/2 c.	22	4	trace	trace	1	14	10	10	107
Radishes, raw	1/2 c.	58	10	trace	trace	2	12	10	14	134
Squash, chayote	1/2 c.	66	16	1	trace	4	13	17	3	99
Squash, scallop	1/2 c.	90	14	1	trace	3	14	25	1	126
Squash, spaghetti	1/2 c.	78	23	1	trace	5	17	11	14	91
Swamp cabbage	1/2 c.	49	10	1	trace	2	26	21	60	139
Turnips, boiled	1/2 c.	78	14	1	trace	4	18	15	39	106
Turnip green, raw	1/2 c.	28	7	trace	trace	2	53	12	11	83
Yambean (jicama)	1/2 c.	60	25	1	trace	5	9	11	4	105

VEGETABLE LIST #2

AVERAGES: Calories: 40 Protein: 1 gm Sodium: 20 mg Potassium: 200 mg Calcium: 27 mg Phosphorus: 36 mg

FOOD ITEM	HOUSEHOLD MEASURE	gm	CAL	gm PRO	m FAT	gm CHO	mg CA	mg P	mg NA	mg K
Artichoke hearts	1/2 c.	84	37	2	trace	9	33	50	55	221
Asparagus, raw	4 spears	58	13	2	trace	2	12	30	1	175
Asparagus, cooked	4 spears	60	16	2	trace	3	15	35	3	159
Beets, cooked	1/2 c.	85	26	1	0	6	9	26	42	266
Broccoli, cooked	1/2 c.	78	32	2	trace	7	24	43	18	251
Burdock root, cooked	1/2 c.	63	55	1	trace	13	31	58	3	225
Carrot, raw	1/2 c.	55	24	1	trace	6	15	24	19	178
Cauliflower, raw	1/2 c.	50	12	1	trace	3	14	23	7	178
Cauliflower, cooked	1/2 c.	76	16	1	trace	3	16	22	10	163
Celeriac, raw	1/2 c.	78	31	1	trace	7	34	90	78	234
Celery, raw	1/2 c.	60	9	trace	trace	2	22	16	53	170
Collards, cooked	1/2 c.	93	30	3	1	6	166	31	34	224
Corn, cooked	1/2 c.	82	78	3	1	19	2	62	9	159
Cress, raw	1/2 c.	25	8	1	trace	1	20	19	4	152
Dock (sorrel), raw	1/2 c.	67	15	1	trace	2	29	42	3	261
Kale, raw	1/2 c.	34	17	1	trace	4	46	19	15	152
Kale, cooked	1/2 c.	65	21	2	trace	4	69	18	13	179
Mixed veg., frozen	1/2 c.	87	47	2	trace	10	22	40	77	197
Okra, boiled	1/2 c.	80	25	2	trace	6	50	45	4	257
Parsley, raw	1/2 c.	30	10	1	trace	2	39	12	12	161
Peas, green, cooked	1/2 c.	82	63	4	trace	12	19	74	25	166

VEGETABLE LIST #2 (continued)

AVERAGES: Calories: 40 Protein: 1 gm Sodium: 20 mg Potassium: 200 mg Calcium: 27 mg Phosphorus: 36 mg

FOOD ITEM	HOUSEHOLD MEASURE	gm	CAL	gm PRO	m FAT	gm CHO	mg CA	mg P	mg NA	mg K
Pepper, chili, raw	1 ea.	45	18	1	trace	4	8	20	3	153
Poi	1/2 c.	120	134	1	trace	33	19	47	14	220
Potato, oiled, no skin	1/2 c.	78	67	1	trace	16	6	31	4	256
Pumpkin, cooked	1/2 c.	122	33	1	trace	8	25	40	4	266
Rutabaga, cooked	1/2 c.	85	29	1	trace	7	36	42	15	244
Spinach, raw	1/2 c.	28	6	1	trace	1	28	14	22	156
Squash, summer, ckd.	1/2 c.	90	18	1	trace	4	24	35	1	173
Squash, zucchini	1/2 c.	90	14	1	trace	4	12	36	2	228
Succotash, cooked	1/2 c.	85	79	4	trace	17	13	59	38	225
Sweet potato, canned	1/2 c.	98	106	1	trace	25	16	25	38	189
Tomato, raw	1/2 c.	90	18	1	trace	4	6	21	8	186
Tomato juice, no salt	1/2 c.	122	21	1	1	5	10	23	12	268

NON-DAIRY PRODUCT LIST

FOOD ITEM	HOUSEHOLD MEASURE	gm	CAL	gm PRO	m FAT	gm CHO	mg CA	mg P	mg NA	mg K
Coffee Rich, liquid	1/4 c.	60	96	0.2	6	11	1	24	24	24
Coffee whiteners, liquid (frozen) avg.	1/4 c.	60	80	0.6	6	7	4	40	48	116
Coffee whiteners, powder, average	2 Tbsp.	12	66	0.6	4	7	trace	48	24	96
Cremora, Borden	2 Tbsp.	12	66	0.6	—	—	—	—	1	10
Dessert Whip, liquid	1/4 c.	60	164	0.6	11	4	—	—	40	20
Imitation sour cream	1/4 c.	56	118	1.4	6	5	2	26	58	92
Mocha Mix	1/4 c.	57	80	0.2	—	—	3	32	29	79
Party Pride Whip, liquid	2 Tbsp.	30	99	0.6	6	—	—	—	13	1
Poly Rich, liquid	1/4 c.	60	88	0.2	6	8	1	20	12	40
Rich's Whip Topping, whipped	1/2 c.	23	63	0	—	—	—	—	13	trace
DESSERTS:										
Gelatin, low Sodium, D'Zerta	1/2 c.	60	8	2.0	0	0	trace	trace	10	50
Gelatin, regular, flavored	1/2 c.	—	71	1.8	0	17	—	—	61	—
Mocha Mix, Frozen Dessert	3/4 c.	—	216	0.6	—	—	—	—	90	—
Sherbet	1/2 c.	96	135	1.1	2	29	51	37	44	90

BEVERAGE LIST

HOUSEHOLD FOOD ITEM	MEASURE	gm	CAL	gm PRO	m FAT	gm CHO	mg CA	mg P	mg NA	mg K
ALCOHOLIC BEVERAGES (use only if approved by Doctor):										
Beer, average	8 oz.	240	101	0.7	0	9	12	72	17	60
Brandy, gin, vodka, rum, whiskey (80 proof)	3 oz.	90	194	—	—	trace	—	—	trace	3
Wine, sweet, dessert	4 oz.	120	164	trace	0	9	8	—	4	92
Wine, sherry	4 oz.	120	164	0.2	0	9	10	—	4	88
Wine, table, average	4 oz.	120	100	0.4	0	5	12	12	4	108
BEVERAGES - Carbonated:										
Bubble-Up	8 oz.	240	90	0	—	22	—	—	33	9
Coca Cola	8 oz.	240	110	0	—	28	—	—	30	2
Gingerale	8 oz.	240	85	0	—	21	—	—	22	9
Hires Root Beer	8 oz.	240	100	0	—	25	—	—	41	3
Pepsi Cola	8 oz.	240	110	0	—	28	—	—	28	9
Royal Crown Cola	8 oz.	240	110	0	—	28	—	—	22	4
Simba	8 oz.	240	90	0	—	22	—	—	40	2
Shasta, club soda	8 oz.	240	0	0	0	0	—	—	131	4
Shasta, sugar free, average	8 oz.	240	1	0	0	trace	—	—	51	4
Shasta, regular, avg.	8 oz.	240	110	0	0	27	—	—	25	4
Shasta, mixes	8 oz.	240	85	0	0	21	—	—	25	4
Tab, sugar free	8 oz.	240	1	0	—	trace	—	—	33	9

BEVERAGE LIST (continued)

HOUSEHOLD FOOD ITEM	MEASURE	gm	CAL	gm PRO	m FAT	gm CHO	mg CA	mg P	mg NA	mg K
BEVERAGES - Coffee, Tea, Bouillon:										
Coffee, regular, instant	1 level tsp.	0.8	1	trace	trace	trace	1	3	1	26
Coffee, freeze dried, instant	1 level tsp.	0.9	1	trace	trace	trace	2	3	1	29
Coffee, instant, prepared from 2 gm powder	6 oz.	180	2	trace	trace	trace	4	7	2	65
Coffee, brewed weak	6 oz.	180	2	trace	trace	trace	2	3	1	112
Postum	6 oz.	180	36	0.6	trace	8	10	87	4	136
Tea	8 oz.	240	2	0.1	0	0	5	4	5	60-130
Bouillon, salted	1 cube	4	5	0.8	trace	trace	—	—	480	4
Bouillon, salted, powder	1 level tsp.	2	2	0.4	trace	trace	—	—	480	2
Awake - Imitation orange juice	4 oz.	124	51	trace	—	13	—	—	5	41
Cranberry juice cocktail	8 oz.	240	164	0.3	0	42	13	8	3	25
Grape tang	8 oz.	240	120	0	0	28	—	—	110	2
Kool Aid, regular	8 oz.	240	100	0	0	25	—	—	1	1
Kool Aid, presweetened	8 oz.	240	90	0	0	23	—	—	1	1
Lemon Tang	8 oz.	240	100	0	0	26	—	—	30	2
Lemonade, frozen, diluted	8 oz.	240	107	0.1	trace	28	2	3	1	40
Limeade, frozen, diluted	8 oz.	240	102	0.1	trace	27	3	3	trace	32
Orange Tang	8 oz.	240	100	0	0	26	—	—	<20	42
Start Instant Breakfast	8 oz.	240	100	0	0	26	—	—	47	47
Tart Orange Tang	8 oz.	240	120	0	0	26	—	—	45	trace

The preceding food charts were provided courtesy of the California Dietetic Association, Los Angeles District.

APPENDIX C
LIST OF COOKBOOKS

Cooking Without a Grain of Salt by E.W. Bagg. Write to: Doubleday and Co., Inc., Bantam Books, New York, NY 10021.

Creative Cooking for Renal Diets and *Creative Cooking for Renal Diabetic Diets* by the Cleveland Clinic Foundation. Write to: Department of Nutrition Services, The Cleveland Clinic Foundation, 9500 Euclid Ave., Cleveland, OH 44106.

Living Salt-Free and Easy by A. Houston-Thorburn and P. Turner. Write to: Douglas-West Publishers, Inc., Signet Books, New York, NY 10021.

Living Well on Dialysis: A Cookbook for Patients and Their Families. A patient education program of the National Kidney Foundation, Inc., developed by the Council on Renal Nutrition. Supported by an educational grant from Amgen, Inc. Contact: The National Kidney Foundation, Inc. (800) 622-9010.

A Nutritional Guide for Persons with Kidney Disease by Cynthia A. DeMotte, M.P.H., R.D. Write to: California Dietetic Association-Los Angeles District, CDA-LAD, P.O. Box 3506, Santa Monica, CA 90403.

The Renal Patient's Guide to Good Eating by Judith A. Curtis. Write to: Charles C. Thomas, Publisher, 2600 South First Street, Springfield, IL 62794-9265.

Recipes for Renal Diets by M. Schumaci. Write to: Saga Food Service, St. Luke's Hospital Center, P.O. Box 479, Utica, NY 13503.

Sodium Controlled Cookbook (Especially for Renal Diets) and *Carbohydrate and Sodium Controlled Cookbook (Especially for Diabetic and CAPD Renal Diets)* by CRN Northern California/Northern Nevada. Write to: Trudy O'Regan, R.D., Washington Hospital, 2000 Mowry Ave., Fremont, CA 94538.

The Gourmet Renal Nutrition Cookbook by Meredith C. Greene, R.D.
Write to: Meredith C. Greene, R.D., c/o Dialysis Unit, Lenox Hill
Hospital, 100 E. 77th St., New York, NY 10021.

The Hillcrest Happy Kidney Cookbook by Hillcrest Renal Disease
Center. Write to: Administrative Director, Hillcrest Renal Disease
Center,1145 S. Utica, Tulsa, OK 74104.

The Renal Family Cookbook ed. by Marian Law, M.A., R.P. Dt. Write
to: American Kidney Fund, 7315 Wisconsin Ave., Suite 203 E,
Bethesda, MD 20814

*Understanding Your Renal Diet, Understanding Your Diet on
CAPD, Understanding Your Renal Diabetic Diet.* Write to:
National Kidney Foundation of Iowa, 8611 Hickman Rd., Des
Moines, IA 50322.

It is important that a patient work together with their dietitian and
physician to select the dietary information that meets their individual
needs.

APPENDIX D
WEIGHTS AND MEASUREMENTS

Dry Measurements	Approximate Conversion
1/4 teaspoon (tsp)	1 gram (gm)
1/2 tsp	2 gm
1 tsp	5 gm
3 tsp = 1 tablespoon (tbsp)	15 gm
2 tbsp = 1 ounce (oz)	30 gm
4 tbsp = 1/4 cup = 2 oz	60 gm
16 tbsp = 1 cup = 8 oz	240 gm

Liquid Measurements	Approximate Conversion to Metric System
2 tbsp = 1 oz	30 milliliters (ml)
1 jigger = 1-1/2 oz	45 ml
1/4 cup = 2 oz	60 ml
1/3 cup = 2-2/3 oz	80 ml
1/2 cup = 4 oz	120 ml
2/3 cup = 5-1/3 oz	160 ml
3/4 cup = 6 oz	180 ml
1 cup = 8 oz	240 ml
2 cups = 16 oz = 1 pint	500 ml
4 cups = 32 oz = 1 quart	1000 ml = 1 liter (L)

NOTE: 1 milliliter (ml) = 1 cubic centimeter (cc)

**APPENDIX E
LIST OF MEDICATIONS**

Type of Drug	Examples of Brand Names	Purpose
Analgesics	Tylenol®	Help relieve pain; some can also reduce fever.
Antibiotics	Cephalosporin Erythromycin Penicillin Tetracycline Vancomycin	Stop the growth of bacteria or kill bacteria.
Phosphate Binders	ALternaGEL® Alucaps® Aludrox® Amphojel® Basaljel® Calcium Acetate Calcium Carbonate	Bind phosphate in intestine to help maintain proper calcium and phosphorus levels in the blood. (See calcium supplements)

	Calcium Hydroxide Oscal® Riopan® Titralac Tums® CALCI-CHEW® CALCI-MIX® NEPHRO-CALCI®	
Potassium Binder	Kayexalate®	Binds potassium in intestine to prevent elevated potassium levels in blood.
Blood Pressure Medications:		
General	Aldomet® Apresoline® Clonidine Hydralazine	Lower blood pressure.
ACE Inhibitors	Capoten® Vasotec®	
Beta Blockers	Inderal® Propranalol	

Calcium Channel Blockers	Procardia ® Nifedipine	
Calcium Supplements	Calcium Carbonate Neo-Calgluconate® Oscal® Titralac Tums® CALCI-CHEW® CALCI-MIX® NEPHRO-CALCI®	Increase the amount of calcium in the blood and body. Also functions as phosphate binders if taken with meals. (See phosphate binders)
Folic Acid	Folic Acid	Needed in production of new red blood cells and helps anemia.
Heart Stimulants	Lanoxin® Digoxin	Make heart beat stronger and slower.
Iron	Fersol® (tablets) Ferrous sulfate InFed (fluid) NEPHRO-FER®	Needed in production of oxygen-carrying molecules in red blood cells. Iron dextran for injection. Often given intravenously.

Male Hormones	Halotestin® Decadurabolin® Depo® Testosterone	Increase red blood cell production by stimulating bone marrow.
Vitamins	Multi-vite (there are many other brands) Nephro-Vite® Nephro-Vite + Fe Z-Bec®	Help maintain normal body functions and supplement vitamins in food.
Vitamin D	Rocaltrol® Calcijex®	Causes body to absorb calcium from food and place it in the bones.
Sleeping Pills and Tranquilizers	Valium® Seconal® Phenobarbital Halcion® Restoril®	Aid in mental and physical relaxation; help to reduce insomnia, restlessness, itching and muscle cramps.

Index

A

American Association of Kidney Patients (AAKP) 94-95, 112, 113, 118, 129, 134

Access device 12, 21, 23, 25

Acetate 15, 18, 30

Acid 3, 15

Acidosis 3

Acid substance 3

Acquired immune deficiency syndrome (AIDS) 133

Acute kidney failure 6, 12, 103

Acute rejection 65-66

Adjustment 22, 65-66, 73-74, 83, 89-90, 94-95, 97-98, 123, 136

Advance directives 139-163
  benefits of 154
  cancelling
  changing 163
  contents of 159-160
  disadvantages of 154-155
  help in preparing 160-161
  learning about 160-161
  preparing 160-161
  rescinding/revoking 163
  teenagers and 159

transplant patients and 158-159
  updating 163

Agent 147

Agent-in-fact 147

AIDS 31, 52, 133

Air detector monitor 20

Alcoholic beverages 82

Allergic 37, 53

Aluminum intoxication 134

Alzheimer's disease 158

American Geriatrics Society, Journal of 161

American Kidney Fund 112-113

American Medical Association, Journal of (JAMA) 161

Analgesics 86

Anemia 4, 49-53, 125

Anemic 21, 33, 38-39, 49-50, 51

Antacid 34, 85

Antibiotics 47, 86

Antibody 133

Anticoagulants 36

Antilymphocyte globulin 67-68

Anti-rejection medications 158

Anxiety 22, 40, 70, 89-90, 92, 93, 95, 96, 132

S

Saline 32

Salt 2, 11, 15, 32, 33, 37, 48, 68, 78-80, 84

Satellite dialysis center 26

Schedule, dialysis
dialysis schedule 18

Scribner Dr. Belding
Dr. Belding Scribner 12

Self-care benefits, Medicare
Medicare self-care benefits 104-105

Self-care dialysis 28, 103-105

Serum hepatitis 30-31

Sexual adjustment 92-93, 96

Sexual function 92-93, 96

Shunt, external 23

Social Security 100, 102, 109-111, 114-115

Social worker 39, 40, 90, 92-93, 95-96, 98, 102-103, 109-110, 112, 113, 119, 121-123

Sodium 2, 32, 33, 36, 70, 73-74, 78-79, 84

Solution exchanges 12

Sterile technique 30, 47

Substituted judgement 146

Success rate 57-58, 66, 69, 117, 124-126

Supplements 33, 41, 86, 88
calcium 34, 86

potassium 2-3, 48, 76-77
vitamins 34, 88

Surrogate decision-maker 145

Swelling 2, 5, 24-25, 32, 37, 65, 67, 79

Systemic lupus erythematosus 8

T

Technicians 39, 40

Temperature monitor 19

Tissue typing 58-59, 60, 62, 107, 126

Toxins 7, 50

Transfusion 21, 31, 38, 39, 51-53, 58

Transplantation 6-7, 9, 12, 17, 40, 57-59, 61, 65, 66, 68-70, 94, 96, 107-108, 117, 125, 133

Transplant patients 158-159

Travel 27, 40, 62, 96, 105, 119, 121-123

Travel agency 123

Treatment 143
goals of 161-163
refusing 140-141
disputes 143-144
patient statements of 162-163

Treatment directive 147-149, 151

U

Ultrafiltration 13, 14, 16, 32
*Understanding Your New
  Life With Dialysis* 123
Uniform Anatomical Gift Act
  61
Unit 39, 53, 83, 97, 109,
  119-123, 133, 134, 137
Urea 3, 36, 38, 74
Uremia 3, 32, 37, 73, 93
Uremic 3, 21
  poisoning 3
  syndrome 3
  toxins 8
Ureter 4, 63
Urethra 4
Urine 2-5, 22, 37, 59, 63,
  76, 81

V

Values history 155-156
Vein 11, 20, 24-25, 63
Venous pressure monitor 19
Veterans benefits 110-111
Vitamin D 4, 34-35, 79, 87
Vitamins 82, 88
Vocational rehabilitation 96-
  98

W

Waste products 2-4, 11, 22,
  23, 35, 38, 43-45, 73, 74-
  75, 93

Weight, dry 37, 82
Weights 84-85
White blood cells 13-14, 69
William B. Dessner Memorial
  Fund, 113
Withdrawing treatment, 142
Withholding treatment, 142